Physician Crisis

Jeffrey N. Weiss

Physician Crisis

Why Physicians Are Leaving Medicine, Why You Should Stay, and How To Be Happy

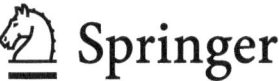 Springer

Jeffrey N. Weiss
Parkland, FL, USA

ISBN 978-3-031-27978-2   ISBN 978-3-031-27979-9   (eBook)
https://doi.org/10.1007/978-3-031-27979-9

This Springer imprint is published by the registered company Springer
Nature Switzerland AG
The registered company address is: Gewerbestrasse 11, 6330 Cham, Switzerland

May the physicians who have the privilege and honor of serving patients be secure in the knowledge that their efforts are noble and respected.

Introduction

John M. is an unemployed mechanic who presented to the Emergency Room with a scratchy left eye. The "scratch" was a corneal ulcer that was caused by an amoeba. The treatment, a $300 per month eye drop. John's answer—"I'm glad I have the other eye." John's Medicaid doesn't pay for the medication. But when the infection progresses, and his eye becomes blind and painful, they will pay to have it removed.

Lois R. presented with vitreous inflammation of the eye. Reticulum Cell Sarcoma was suspected. Her Primary Care Physician (PCP) refused to order an MRI because he never heard of the condition. Despite multiple telephone calls and faxed information, he refused to order the test. Six months later, she presented to the emergency room with a convulsion and subsequently died of reticulum cell sarcoma. The patient was on an HMO and her PCP receives a financial bonus by "containing expenses."

Linda Peeno, M.D., was a medical reviewer for Humana and Medical Director at Blue Cross/Blue Shield Health Plans. On May 30, 1996, she testified before Congress that HMOs drive profits through denial of care.

She said:

"I wish to begin by making a public confession: In the spring of 1987, as a physician, I caused the death of a man. Although this was known to many people, I have not been taken before any court of law or called to account for this in any professional or public forum. In fact, just the opposite occurred: I was 'rewarded' for this. It bought me an improved reputation in my job, and contributed to my advancement afterwards. Not only did I demonstrate I could indeed do what was expected of me, I exemplified the 'good' company doctor: I saved a half million dollars.

I contend that 'managed care,' as we currently know it, is inherently unethical in its organization and operation. Furthermore, I maintain that we have an industry which can exist only through flagrant ethical violations against individuals and the public."

The essence of her statement is that private companies can do things that the government is not allowed to do. And since the government and politicians benefit from the HMO actions, whether they are egregious or not, they will do little to curb the problems.

Robert J's left leg was amputated due to diabetes. Medicaid would not pay for a prosthesis. He awoke at night to find rats chewing at his bloody stump.

Rabbi Grossman was diabetic. He could not afford his insulin. He contacted the insulin manufacturer for help, and they provided him with a 3-month supply of insulin. After the 3month supply was used up, he was on his own.

Dr. W. billed Blue Cross of Florida. He never got paid because they said they never received the claims. He resent them through Certified Mail, Return Receipt Requested. No payment. When he called Blue Cross, they said that the person who signed for the letters no longer worked there. He resent the information through Registered Mail. Ten months later, he received a payment. The amount was less than he should have received, and he was advised to bill the patient for the balance.

A doctor complained to the HMO that patients who needed cataract surgery were being sent for eyeglasses. The HMO cancelled the doctor's contract. The patients still didn't receive cataract surgery. Unfortunately, many of the patients were unsophisticated and incapable of challenging the HMO's decisions.

These are only a paltry few of the many, many stories of the failure of the US healthcare system. Patients and physicians are pawns in a system dominated by the government, insurance companies, hospital companies, and drug companies.

There is too much money at stake to make significant and meaningful changes. And our politicians are beholden to their lobbyists who support their campaigns and may give them high paying jobs when they leave office.

As long as the majority of people have reasonable medical coverage, there is no incentive to change. Politicians will always obtain the best healthcare for themselves. Physicians need to make the best of a broken system. Understanding what is going on is the first step in dealing with the problem.

Contents

Chapter 1
The Nature of the Problem

A September 2022 article by Lorna Collier in "Healthgrades for Professionals" is entitled "7 Reasons Doctors Are Leaving Medicine."

Approximately 16,000 practices closed in 2020 due to the COVID-19 pandemic. But an earlier 2018 study found that 54% of physicians were considering retirement by 2023. Why?

1.1 Burnout

Forty-seven percent of doctors report burnout due to bureaucracy, lack of respect, and too many work hours. Female doctors report a higher burnout rate (56%) than male colleagues (41%). Critical care and emergency medicine are the top "burned out" specialties. Disturbingly, 13% of physicians felt suicidal, and 1% have already attempted suicide.

1.2 Bureaucracy

Sixty percent of physicians cited bureaucracy as the number one reason for burnout in a 2022 Medscape survey. Twenty-five percent of physician time was spent on nonclinical paperwork, a 2016 report found.

© The Author(s), under exclusive license to Springer Nature Switzerland AG 2023
J. N. Weiss, *Physician Crisis*,
https://doi.org/10.1007/978-3-031-27979-9_1

1.3   Loss of Independence

A 2022 study by Physicians Advocacy Institute found that 74% of physicians work for a corporate entity or are employed by a hospital. Even a group practice may now be owned by a private equity group. Administrators rather than physicians dictate case load based on profit, not on best patient care.

1.4   Electronic Medical Records (EMR)

Many surveys have listed that EMR has a prominent cause of physician dissatisfaction. The doctor spends time looking at a computer screen rather than the patient. One hour of patient care translates into 2 h of time spent on EMR. Much of the information is unnecessary, redundant and is only used to satisfy insurance billing requirements. Important information is lost within the meaningless data.

1.5   Long Hours

Thirty-four percent of physicians cited long work hours as the reason for burnout in a Medscape 2022 report. Forty percent of female doctors and less than 5% of male doctors reported that they quit medicine due to family reasons.

1.6   Low Income

Twenty-eight percent of physicians cited low pay causing burnout in a Medscape 2022 survey. It is difficult for physicians in low paying specialties, or low paying jobs, to pay student loans or malpractice premiums.

1.7   Patient Bullying

The COVD-19 pandemic has increased the bullying and verbal abuse by patients who do not believe that there is a pandemic, and refuse vaccination. They are accusing physicians of not acting in the patient's best interests but rather as a tool of drug companies.

A recent article in Mayo Clinic Proceedings: Innovation, Quality & Outcomes, "COVID-Related Stress and Work Intentions in a Sample of U.S. Health Care Workers" found that 20% of physicians report that they will leave their current practice within 2 years and 33% state that they will reduce their working hours within the next year.

The U.S. spends more money on healthcare than any other nation in the world. The gross domestic product share of healthcare is estimated at 18% and is rising. Waste accounts for approximately 30% of the total. U.S. healthcare spending in 2019 is projected at $3.82 trillion dollars. The annual cost of wasteful spending from pharmaceutical pricing failure is estimated at approximately $230–$240 billion. New high-cost specialty drugs, i.e., cancer, will exceed 50% of pharmaceutical spending.

The Institute of Medicine and Berwick and Hackbarth identified six medical waste domains. A 2019 study reviewed 54 peer-reviewed publications, government reports, and gray literature reports. Estimated total annual costs of waste were $760 billion–$935 billion.

In 2019, 9.2% of the U.S. population was uninsured. The range was from a low in Massachusetts, 3%, to a high of 18.4% in Texas. In 2020, medical spending per person was $11,945, more than $4000 greater than any other high-income country. Yet the U.S. ranks #11 in population health.

Health care in 11 high-income countries was analyzed. Seventy one performance measures across five domains were analyzed: access to care, care process, administrative efficiency, equity, and health care outcomes. The data was obtained from the Organization for Economic Cooperation and Development, the World Health Organization, and from Commonwealth Fund international surveys. Of the 11 countries, the U.S. ranked last, despite spending far more of its GDP on health care. The U.S. was also last on access to care, administrative efficiency, equity, and outcomes, but second on measures of care process.

What do the higher-ranking countries provide that the U.S. does not? There are four features:

1. Universal coverage and the removal of cost barriers
2. An investment in primary care available to everyone
3. Less administrative burden
4. Investment in social services

The Roman lawyer Cicero (106–43 BC) in his treatise, "On Moral Duties," warned politicians to serve the interest of those they represent, rather than their own private interests. Unfortunately, politician's goals are to get, and stay elected, not to serve the public good. And elections require a great deal of money. 40% of a politician's time is spent raising money for election. Who provides this money? Large lobbying groups. We have the best government that money can buy. Too many groups are making too much money at the expense of the public health.

There are certain realities that must be acknowledged. Politician's opinions change with the wind. Staunch Republicans who were against abortion were changing their tune following the overturning of Roe v. Wade and the resulting popular backlash. They want to get elected.

Large companies, like pharmaceutical companies, hospital chains, and insurance companies, have large lobbies and a lot of money to fund political campaigns. As long as a majority of the population are somewhat satisfied with their healthcare, there is no incentive to change.

In a free market economy, the government has little power to impose changes. The government can pile on more regulations adding to the cost of doing business, but is incapable of removing additional expenses. Their answer, reduce payments. It takes work to decrease costs, and in many cases, the government benefits from the additional funds. It takes no work, intelligence, or effort to reduce everyone else's payments, i.e., physicians, by a certain percentage and justify the action by a nonsensical explanation.

The government can also spend more money on feeding the system. They can extend healthcare to the uninsured by subsidizing care. They can reimburse patients for pharmaceuticals. Could they regulate health insurance companies like utilities? In effect they now do, forcing insurance companies to return premiums when a particular percentage of their health care dollars is not "spent on health care."

Medicare pays below the cost of care. They justify this by stating that many hospitals and physicians are "not efficient." Is the government the arbiter of efficiency? Do they pay less for the trucks they purchase because the manufacturer could be more efficient? And how do they define "efficient?" In Florida, private health care plans pay physicians from 60% to 80% of Medicare rates. Physicians are barely surviving.

In a laissez-faire capitalist system with a two major party-political system that depends on raising money to get elected, unrestricted political donations, and extensive lobbying by major groups, the government can tweak but not dismantle the present system. There is no point in recommending the impossible. In this book, I am going to suggest how physicians can successfully deal with the present system. Let us investigate the various factors in healthcare by going back to the beginning, the making of a doctor.

Suggested Readings

Association of American Medical Colleges. Why women leave medicine. 2019. https://www.aamc.org/news-insights/why-women-leave-medicine.

Bankrate. What is the average medical school debt? 2022. https://www.bankrate.com/loans/student-loans/average-medical-school-debt/.

Berwick DM, Hackbarth AD. Eliminating waste in US Health Care. JAMA. 2012;307(14):1513–6. https://doi.org/10.1001/jama.2012.362.

Care ATC. 5 Reasons Why Physicians Are Leaving the Practice (And Where They Want to Go). n.d. https://www.careatc.com/ehs/5-reasons-why-physicians-are-leaving-the-practice-and-where-they-want-to-go.

Fierce Healthcare. Physicians' departure from private practice has accelerated since 2018, AMA says. 2021. https://www.fiercehealth-care.com/practices/physicians-departure-from-private-practice-has-accelerated-since-2018-ama-says.

Hanson M. Average medical student debt. Education Data. 2022. https://educationdata.org/average-medical-school-debt.

KHN. Institute of medicine. https://khn.org/morning-breakout/iom-report/. Accessed 9 June 2022.

Mitchell Louis. Private equity is ruining American healthcare–physicians, patients lose when PE takes over; it's time to take medicine back. MedPage Today. 2021. https://www.medpagetoday.com/opinion/second-opinions/93615.

Medscape. Why doctors are leaving the profession. Onyx MD. https://www.onyxmd.com/about-onyx-md/blog/why-doctors-are-leaving-the-profession/Medscape Physician Compensation Report 2020. https://www.medscape.com/slideshow/2020-compensation-overview-6012684#18.

Medscape. 'Death by 1000 cuts': medscape national physician burnout & suicide report 2021a. https://www.medscape.com/slideshow/2021-lifestyle-burnout-6013456.

Medscape. Medscape residents salary & debt report 2021b. https://www.medscape.com/slideshow/2021-residents-salary-debt-report-6014074#3.

Medscape. Physician burnout and depression: stress, anxiety and anger. 2022. https://www.medscape.com/slideshow/2022-lifestyle-burnout-6014664#4.

Gretchen Morgenson and Emmanuelle Saliba. Private equity firms now control many hospitals, ERs and nursing homes. Is it good for health care? NBC News. 2020. https://www.nbcnews.com/health/health-care/private-equity-firms-now-control-many-hospitals-ers-nursing-homes-n1203161.

Kevin B. O'Reilly. New research links hard-to-use EHRs and physician burnout. American Medical Association. 2019. https://www.ama-assn.org/practice-management/digital/new-research-links-hard-use-ehrs-and-physician-burnout.

Physicians Advocacy Institute. COVID 19's impact on acquisitions of physicians practices and physician employment 2019-2021. 2022. http://www.physiciansadvocacyinstitute.org/Portals/0/assets/docs/PAI-Research/PAI%20Avalere%20Physician%20Employment%20Trends%20Study%202019-21%20Final.pdf?ver=ksWkgjKXB_yZfImFdXlvGg%3d%3d.

Shanafelt TD, Boone S, Tan L, et al. Burnout and satisfaction with work-life balance among US physicians relative to the general US Population. Arch Intern Med. 2012;172(18):1377–85. https://doi.org/10.1001/archinternmed.2012.3199.

Shrank WH, Rogstad TL, Parekh N. Waste in the US health care system: estimated costs and potential for savings. JAMA. 2019;322(15):1501–9. https://doi.org/10.1001/jama.2019.13978.

The Physicians Foundation. 2020 survey of America's physicians: the COVID-19 impact edition. 2020. https://physiciansfoundation.org/wp-content/uploads/2020/08/20-1278-Merritt-Hawkins-2020-Physicians-Foundation-Survey.6.pdf.

Thornell C. Physicians report that organizational and technology changes are among the biggest burnout factors. Athena. Health. 2021; https://www.athenahealth.com/knowledge-hub/clinical-trends/physicians-report-organizational-technology-changes-among-biggest-burnout-factors

Chapter 2
Getting into Medical School

As of 2022, there were 155 accredited medical schools in the U.S.

2.1 2022 Admissions

During the 2021–2022 admission cycle, 22,666 of the 62,443 (approximately 36%) students who applied matriculated into a medical school. From 2013 to 2022, female medical school applicants increased from 46.2% to 56.8% and in the 2021–2022 academic year, more women applied to medical school than men by 13.6%.

The Association of American Medical Colleges reports that there has been a 25% increase in the number of applicants in late 2020 compared to 2019. The normal year to year growth is approximately 3%. The large increase in applicants is felt to be due to the COVID-19 pandemic. This mirrors the increase in applications to the military after 9/11.

At the ten top medical schools, the admission rate is 2.6% or less. Two of the top ten medical schools, New York University and the Kaiser Permanente Bernard J. Tyson School of Medicine offer free tuition.

© The Author(s), under exclusive license to Springer Nature Switzerland AG 2023

J. N. Weiss, *Physician Crisis*,
https://doi.org/10.1007/978-3-031-27979-9_2

Why do people wish to become a doctor?

1. Respected profession
2. Always needed
3. Calling: It's who you are

What are the problems with becoming a doctor?

1. Less physician autonomy—decrease in private practice opportunities. Physicians working for large corporations
2. Increasing liability
3. Interference from state legislatures on the practice of medicine and increased threat of legal attacks and liability
4. Increased bureaucracy
5. Electronic medical records—Charting requirements and documenting. Doctors have become clerical workers and administrators. Notes designed for insurance companies and government and not efficient care of patients. Physicians spend more time with the computer than with the patient. Emergency room doctors have more charting than neurosurgeons, and they burn out faster
6. Low reimbursements
7. High medical school debt
8. Competition from ancillary health care groups—nurse practitioners, optometrists, etc.
9. Added regulations and billing requirements

Suggested Reading

Hartstein L. Surprising medical school statistics (2022)–Inspira Advantage. 2022. https://www.inspiraadvantage.com/blog/surprising-medical-school-statistics-2022. Accessed 8 June 2022.

U.S. News and World Reports. What are the hardest medical schools to get into? 2022. https://www.usnews.com/best-graduate-schools/top-medical-schools/hardest-to-get-into-rankings. Accessed 7 July 2022.

Chapter 3
Financing Medical School

The Association of American Medical Colleges (AAMC) reports that the Class of 2021 held a median medical school debt of $200,000, exclusive of undergraduate debt. Seventy-four percent of students had an education debt. Fourteen percent of students at public medical school held at least $300,000 in medical and undergraduate debt.

The average cost to attend an in-state public institution was $38,947, inclusive of tuition, fees, and health insurance.

The average medical school debt at a private medical school is $218,746. Seventy percent of graduates had education debt, twenty-seven percent of respondents held medical and undergraduate debt of $300,000.

Private institutions—average of $61,023 tuition per year.

New York University, Cleveland Clinic, and Kaiser Permanente have programs to waive medical school tuition. Ancillary living and administrative expenses are not covered.

3.1   How Much Will You Earn?

The Association of American Medical Colleges (AAMC)— average intern salary $57,863.

© The Author(s), under exclusive license to Springer Nature   11
Switzerland AG 2023
J. N. Weiss, *Physician Crisis*,
https://doi.org/10.1007/978-3-031-27979-9_3

Bureau of Labor Statistics—median annual wages of M.D. post residency or fellowship is at least $208,000. Anesthesiologist—average salary of $331,190.

Physician Compensation Report—Medscape 2022.

How Much Did Physicians Earn Overall?

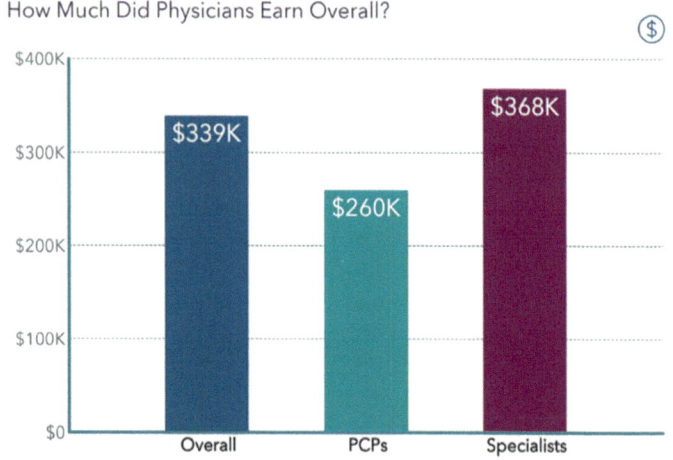

Average Annual Physician Compensation (by Specialty)

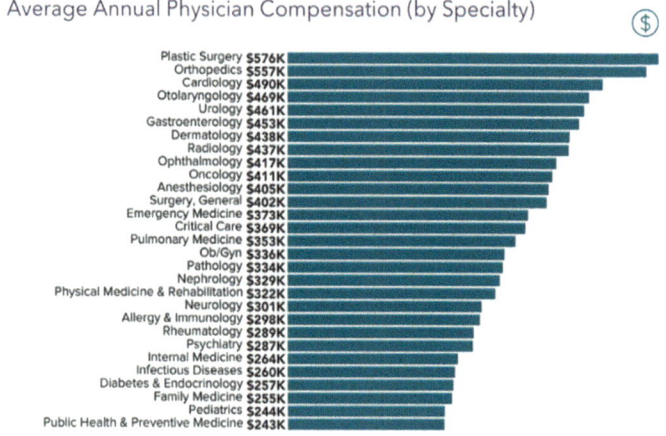

3.2   Doximity Survey

Highest salaries.

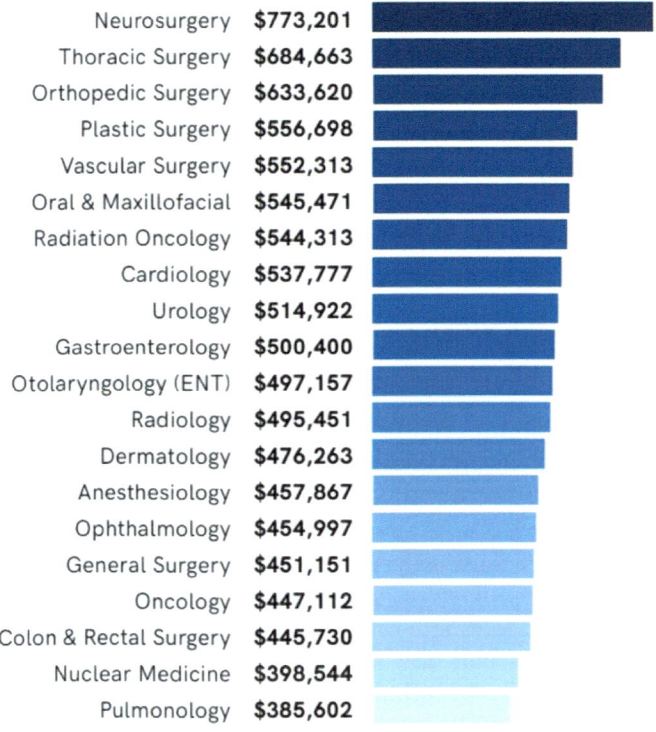

Neurosurgery	**$773,201**
Thoracic Surgery	**$684,663**
Orthopedic Surgery	**$633,620**
Plastic Surgery	**$556,698**
Vascular Surgery	**$552,313**
Oral & Maxillofacial	**$545,471**
Radiation Oncology	**$544,313**
Cardiology	**$537,777**
Urology	**$514,922**
Gastroenterology	**$500,400**
Otolaryngology (ENT)	**$497,157**
Radiology	**$495,451**
Dermatology	**$476,263**
Anesthesiology	**$457,867**
Ophthalmology	**$454,997**
General Surgery	**$451,151**
Oncology	**$447,112**
Colon & Rectal Surgery	**$445,730**
Nuclear Medicine	**$398,544**
Pulmonology	**$385,602**

3.3   Lowest Salaries

Ped. Infectious Disease	**$210,844**
Ped. Rheumatology	**$216,969**
Ped. Endocrinology	**$220,358**
Ped. Hematology & Onc.	**$238,783**
Ped. Nephrology	**$247,861**
Pediatrics	**$251,657**
Medical Genetics	**$254,128**
Ped. Pulmonology	**$263,106**
Medicine/Pediatrics	**$264,254**
Preventive Medicine	**$264,539**
Geriatrics	**$268,861**
Endocrinology	**$270,116**
Family Medicine	**$273,865**
Child Neurology	**$276,420**
Ped. Emergency Medicine	**$280,373**
Infectious Disease	**$294,768**
Internal Medicine	**$295,607**
Ped. Gastroenterology	**$295,751**
Rheumatology	**$303,511**
Occupational Medicine	**$310,934**

Note that despite the COVID-19 pandemic, infectious disease specialists are low paid. Consequently, infectious disease residencies are reporting a decrease in the number of applicants. This does not portend well for the next pandemic.

Suggested Reading

Medical School Insiders. https://medschoolinsiders.com. Accessed 6th April, 2022.

The Association of American Medical Colleges. https://www.aamc.org/. Accessed 6th April, 2022.

Chapter 4
Medical School Curriculum

4.1 How Has the Medical School Curriculum Changed Over the Years?

New additions to the curriculum:

1. Cost consciousness
2. Gun violence
3. Nutrition
4. Opioids and addiction medicine

There has been a decrease in the number of traditional lectures and an increase in collaborative instruction. There has been a decrease in the amount of time spent in the laboratory. USMLE examination Step 1 is now pass/fail, instead of graded.

The medical school application process evaluation has changed.

New methods—personal characteristics, how well the applicant works in teams, how they interact with diverse people, the ability to be resilient, adapt to different situations, and ability to think critically.

The Association of American Medical Colleges (AAMC)—sponsored Medical College Admission Test (MCAT), added two new sections covering critical thinking as well as behavioral and social sciences, in addition to the standard biologic and physical science, and verbal reasoning, among other areas.

© The Author(s), under exclusive license to Springer Nature Switzerland AG 2023
J. N. Weiss, *Physician Crisis*,
https://doi.org/10.1007/978-3-031-27979-9_4

Multiple mini-interviews or MMI uses a series of short scenarios to assess a candidate's soft skills and is supposedly more effective than a traditional interview.

There is a desire to recruit a diverse student body with an interest in caring for underserved populations—including programs and policies for minorities underrepresented in medicine, students from disadvantaged backgrounds, and students from rural and underserved communities.

The emphasis has changed from treating acute to chronic conditions, and problems related to aging. New topics like geriatrics, pain management and palliative care, disease prevention, health promotion, addiction, communication skills, social determinants of health emergency preparedness, and medical informatics have been added to the core curriculum.

Some schools require students to perform nonmedical community service.

System problem-based learning—which consists of 6–10 students and a physician, who go through a hypothetical patient scenario.

Team based learning—several smaller simultaneous groups with one teacher.

Flipped classroom—students study at home, and class is reserved for questions and hands on work.

4.2   Curriculum Change in Medical Schools

Liaison Committee on Medical Education (LCME) Annual Medical School Questionnaire Part II 2017–2018

19.1%	A curriculum change has been instituted in the last 3 years
30.6%	A curriculum change is in the process (not completed) in the last 3 years
34.7%	A curriculum change is planned
15.7%	No curriculum change is planned

Suggested Reading

Association of American Medical Colleges. How medical education is changing. https://www.aamc.org/system/files/c/2/472906-howmedicaleducationischanging.pdf.

Blood AD, Farnan JM, Fitz-William W. Curriculum changes and trends 2010–2020: a focused national review using the AAMC curriculum inventory and the LCME annual medical school questionnaire part II. Acad Med. 2020;95(9S A Snapshot of Medical Student Education in the United States and Canada: Reports From 145 Schools):S5–S14. https://doi.org/10.1097/ACM.0000000000003484. PMID: 33626633 Review.

Boston University Chobanian & Avedisian School of Medicine. Curriculum. https://www.bumc.bu.edu/busm/admissions/curriculum/. Accessed 5 July 2022.

Chapter 5
Post Medical School Graduate Training

Major teaching hospital settings train 74% of residents. This number is decreasing as for-profit and non-profit hospital chains now administer their own residency programs as a means to bolster personnel at a much lower cost than by hiring trained staff. Is this residency as good as a traditional program at a large public hospital? Will the attending physicians be as good? Will the student see the full breath of medical diagnosis and treatments? Probably not, but the question is, is all that necessary?

Most physicians treat the most common conditions, just like most airline pilots are competent. But when there is an emergency, what happens then? Sully Sullenberger, of "the Miracle on the Hudson," said at a Congressional hearing that the average airline pilot does not have the training nor the experience to handle a significant emergency. Nor would a physician not subject to the most rigorous training.

Residency is an important educational program generally lasting from 3 to 7 years after obtaining the M.D. degree. There should be a gradual increase in responsibility with decreasing levels of faculty supervision.

There is a pilot project of time to competency-based advancement in order to shorten the required time for residency. The consequence of this action will be that there are more physicians, but they will not be as well trained or

J. N. Weiss, *Physician Crisis*,
https://doi.org/10.1007/978-3-031-27979-9_5

experienced as those physicians who were products of the traditional system.

Who generates the new performance metrics? Not physicians.

Teams, improving population health, continuous quality improvement in care delivery are the new mantras.

But who determines what improvement in quality means? Not physicians.

There is another issue:

Residency programs using Electronic Residency Application Service software programs may automatically filter out low test scoring or international students. There are as many as 10,000 chronically unmatched doctors in the U.S. The National Resident Matching Program reports a 94% match rate for U.S. trained medical students, but only 61% for foreign medical school graduates.

In 2020, the Association of American Medical Colleges reported that there would be a physician shortage of 54,100–139,000 physicians by 2033. Yet there is a pool of new physicians who because they have not completed a residency are unable to qualify for state licensure.

Suggested Reading

Koea J, Rahiri JL, Ronald M. Affirmative action programs in post-graduate medical and surgical training: a narrative review. Med Educ. 2021;55(3):309–16. https://doi.org/10.1111/medu.14350. Epub 2020 Sep 7.

Sheng J, Manjunath S, Michael M, et al. Integrating handover curricula in medical school. Clin Teach. 2020;17(6):661–8. https://doi.org/10.1111/tct.13181. Epub 2020 Jul 3

Chapter 6
Jobs

It has become increasingly difficult to start a private practice. The regulatory burdens, the cost of Electronic Medical Records (EMR) and equipment is prohibitive for one physician to afford. Physicians are joining group practices, whether single specialty or multispecialty practices, or being employed by hospitals. The freedom of owning and building your own practice, based upon your abilities, is severely limited.

6.1 Hospital Employment

Physicians who sell their practice to a hospital corporation are initially happy. The payout is generous, but their attitude changes over time. Corporate mechanisms are instituted, staffing is reduced, and the physician works harder without the control to influence the work environment. The contract may last 2 years, then the office may be closed and/or the physician is terminated. The patients belong to the hospital, and they can employ another new physician at a lower cost than the old one.

During the COVID-19 pandemic, the hospitalists at my hospital were hailed as heroes. As the pandemic began to wind down, the hospital, (a for-profit corporation), reduced

© The Author(s), under exclusive license to Springer Nature Switzerland AG 2023
J. N. Weiss, *Physician Crisis*,
https://doi.org/10.1007/978-3-031-27979-9_6

their salaries by 30%. Several quit, and as there were no new hires, the remaining hospitalists were forced to work much harder.

More recently, the Florida for-profit hospital has taken the private patients of physicians and assigned them to their own hospitalists. This has resulted in a lawsuit. Next, that same hospital tried to change the hospital bylaws to allow hospital employed radiologists in another state to vote in Florida. This would dilute the vote of the local physicians with those of out of state hospital employees. This action has resulted in another lawsuit.

The physician owned surgicenter where I work was recently sold to another large for-profit hospital chain. The physicians made a lot of money selling their stock to the new owner. But we are paying for it now. The number of staff were cut, and the remaining employees had their salaries reduced. Less people are doing more work, and the place has become much less efficient and surgeon friendly. Both employee and physician moral have suffered. I left as a result.

Almost without exception, in my experience, physicians working at a for-profit hospital corporation are unhappy, at least in South Florida, where I work.

You have to follow the money. Administrators are typically short-term positions at any for-profit hospital. They have to make their numbers, or in other words, profits. If they do, they receive a bonus and perhaps a promotion to a larger hospital. Your happiness isn't their concern. You are only a means to an end.

A January 2022 article by the American Medical Association (AMA) offered suggestions to prevent the upcoming doctor resignation. Their solutions, to be implemented by administration, include:

- Better communication
- Child care
- Rapid training when physicians are sent to unfamiliar situations

To prevent burnout, administrators can:

- Provide personal protective equipment
- Create better hospital environment
- Provide confidential mental health services
- Reduce work overload
- Improve practice efficiency and organizational culture

I laughed when I read this list. They should have also listed frequent visits from the "tooth fairy." The odds of having any of these things are the same. With due respect to the AMA, they are trying, but have no power to affect these changes. That is why Amazon and Starbucks employees are forming unions, to have a voice in negotiating with the corporations.

The activities that the AMA suggest costs money, while administrators want to make money, not spend it on non-incoming producing activities. In fairness to administrators, they are also caught between a peripatetic congress that only wants to lower reimbursement and insurance companies that want to do the same. They are the elephants, and the physicians are the ants. That is why if you want to be happy in practicing medicine in the U.S. you must take control of your own destiny, not rely on the good will and munificence of others who do not have the same goals and interests as you.

Suggested Reading

1. Hallak A, Barnett ME, Hamburg N, Ratchford EV. SVM communications: finding a job after fellowship–a conversation with (gainfully employed) experts. Vasc Med. 2022;27(3):317–9. https://doi.org/10.1177/1358863X221096181.
2. Turin TC, Chowdhury N, Ekpekurede M, et al. Alternative career pathways for international medical graduates towards job market integration: a literature review. Int J Med Educ. 2021;12:45–63. https://doi.org/10.5116/ijme.606a.e83d. PMID: 33839694; PMCID: PMC8415394.

Chapter 7
Electronic Medical Records (EMR)

Why are there no more steam locomotives running on the rails of any modern railroad? Because they were notoriously inefficient, for each hour on the rails, they spent 2 h in the shop. Much like EMR today. For each hour of patient care, the physician must spend 2 h entering data, much like a secretary, except, unlike the secretary, the time the physician spends on entering data in an EMR is not compensated.

The problem is much of the information is repetitive nonsense designed for billing insurance companies or for compliance with government regulations. Important patient care information is mixed with and often hidden within the unimportant information. The record is supposed to reflect what was actually done. But when much of the record is boilerplate, and repetitive, just because it is written doesn't mean it was actually done. And a mistake is memorialized and may be carried through the record for years. A woman patient with a normal prostate examination? A male with a negative pregnancy test? Endless pages of "WNL" when none of the examination was actually performed (WNL = We Never Looked). Ancillary staff performing testing and exams but "signed" by the physician who may or may not have ever seen the patient.

You don't have to be a genius to understand that the presence of more guns leads to more shootings, more opioid pre-

J. N. Weiss, *Physician Crisis*,
https://doi.org/10.1007/978-3-031-27979-9_7

scriptions lead to more deaths, and the more time a physician spends looking at the computer, the less time the physician has for patient care.

At a particular hospital, the administration times how long a physician spends with the patient. They are able to do this by a chip within the physician's identification badge. Billing is paramount in this for-profit hospital so most of the time is spent looking at the screen. Because the physician does not have enough time to do a reasonable examination, many of the patients are admitted to the hospital for simple things and with the wrong diagnosis.

In 2016 Study—Physicians spend about 2 h doing computer work for each hour spent with a patient, regardless of the company manufacturing the computer software. Physicians spend ½ their patient time looking at a computer screen.

Computer work continued after hours, with the average family physician now working 11½ h per day. Forty percent of physicians report depression, 7% suicidal thinking, almost double the rate of the general working population.

Paper charts were brief, notes were to the point, and important information was clearly visible. Nor could they be hacked in data breaches. Now the patient's hobbies, and many irrelevant issues including each code, a justification for why each test was ordered, how much time was supposedly spent, and by whom, assumes the same prominence, and is mixed in with the important information. The lists are deficient, long, and redundant. Physicians must hunt through pages and pages of non-important information needed for the insurance company and government billing and compliance, to find what is important.

Ordering a test used to be one click on a keyboard, now its 11 clicks. Pointless, meaningless work reduces the quality of patient care and the quality of being a physician. This is wasted and uncompensated time, and causing older, and more experienced physicians to leave medicine.

Suggested Reading

Evans RS. Electronic health records: then, now, and in the future. Yearb Med Inform. 2016;Suppl 1(Suppl 1):S48–61. https://doi.org/10.15265/IYS-2016-s006. PMID: 27199197; PMCID: PMC5171496.

Gawande A. Why doctors hate their computers|The New Yorker. 2018.   https://www.newyorker.com/magazine/2018/11/12/why-doctors-hate-their-computers.

Graber ML, Byrne C, Johnston D. The impact of electronic health records on diagnosis. Diagnosis (Berl). 2017;4(4):211–23. https://doi.org/10.1515/dx-2017-0012.

Janett RS, Yeracaris PP. Electronic medical Records in the American Health System: challenges and lessons learned. Cien Saude Colet. 2020;25(4):1293–304. https://doi.org/10.1590/1413-81232020254.28922019. Epub 2019 Oct 22.

Shenoy A, Appel JM. Safeguarding confidentiality in electronic health records. Camb Q Healthc Ethics. 2017;26(2):337–41. https://doi.org/10.1017/S0963180116000931.

Chapter 8
"Burnout"

Christina Maslach, a Berkeley psychologist defines "burnout" as emotional exhaustion, a sense of personal ineffectiveness, and depersonalization or a cynical instrumental attitude toward others. The Maslach Burnout Inventory is a 22 question survey that has been used to track workers emotional well-being.

In 2011, 46% of physicians reported one burnout symptom. In 2014, that number had increased to 54%. As a result, physicians switched to part-time work, or left practice altogether.

It is interesting that emergency physicians have a better than average work-life balance but had the highest burnout scores as compared to neurosurgeons, who had poor work-life balance but lower burnout levels. What could account for these results? A Mayo clinic study determined that the strongest predictor of burnout was, you guessed it, time spent doing computer documentation.

Endless and meaningless documentation fills the patient chart. It is difficult to separate the wheat from the chaff. Physicians became disconnected from one another. The work of office assistants has been transferred to the doctors. They became their own secretaries, in addition to their roles as physicians. Office assistants do not have access to the physician computer screens. And when there is an error, it is very

© The Author(s), under exclusive license to Springer Nature Switzerland AG 2023
J. N. Weiss, *Physician Crisis*,
https://doi.org/10.1007/978-3-031-27979-9_8

difficult to fix, so errors are propagated from screen to screen till time immemorial.

The anticipated benefits of electronic medical records are the portability between offices and hospitals. But, do you really want your ear nose and throat doctor to know you had an STD? However, with HIPPA, privacy concerns, data breaches and hacking, liability, and the fact that office-based systems don't connect with hospital systems, and different hospitals don't share information, this is just a pipe dream.

Large amounts of data do have value. And there is an advantage for patients to be allowed access to their medical information. But to all their medical information? Can they truly understand and correctly interpret their clinical course? Can a doctor record that the patient is an alcoholic, or is married to a woman, but having sex with men, in the medical record that other physicians, including his wife's physician, may see?

Big data can be useful to analyze trends and for research purposes. But at the present time, it is driving physicians out of practice. Is the EMR for medical or billing purposes? For health care, or liability protection? Reducing programs to the important medical information, and eliminating the meaningless excess would help. So would standard pre-programmed orders for individual physicians.

And what happens once the physician is already on one vendor's EMR and they raise their prices, or even go out of business, and there is no longer any support? Individual office-based EMR systems can cost more than $50,000 to install, with a $10,000 per year support fee. Hospital systems can cost more than $500,000 to install, with a $100,000 per year support fee.

Physician reimbursements have been steadily declining. Any reason is used to justify the decrease in reimbursement, and if none is available, a reason is made up. Reimbursement for vitrectomy surgery is lower than the cost of equipment used to perform the surgery. The reimbursement is as low as whatever they can get away with. It is easy to lower reimbursement and add on unfunded mandates, but it takes effort to determine why something is so expensive and then work on removing the unnecessary regulations, bureaucracy, and waste, that keep the costs high.

Frivolous malpractice claims, and complicated medical trials in front of an uneducated jury with automatic sympathies to the claimants, raise the cost of medical care. Unfortunately, when trial lawyers are legislators, and their organization has a large lobby, there is a vested interest in keeping the system as it is.

One answer to the EMR problem has been the medical scribe. This person enters into the computer what the physician dictates. Paper charts were inefficient, but cheap, and now because of computer issues, we need to hire more people. Scribes are minimally trained and underpaid. Their error rates in recording data range between 24% and 50%. But at least the physician can spend more time with the patient, rather than with the computer screen. A 2015 study demonstrated a 36% reduction in physician computer time with a similar increase in time spent with the patient. But there was no increase in job satisfaction. Why? Because the hospital scheduled more patients with the doctor since he/she now had more "free time."

Deming developed a quality system in which there was a collaborative effort between members of the team to improve patient quality. In Florida, in order to maintain your medical license, all physicians must take a medical-errors course. And every year the instructors show the same slide, that of an Indy 500 pit crew working as a team to get the car on the road. But what relevance does this have to physicians? We have no say in the hospital hiring or firing process. The hospital hires the minimum number of people at the lowest cost. Certainly, this is not like a racing pit crew. The physician may be the "Captain of the Ship," but only for liability purposes, he is the toothless tiger without any true power in making the system work better.

Suggested Reading

Deming WE. The new economics: for industry, government, education. Cambridge: MIT Press; 2000. ISBN 978-0-262-54116-9.

Deming WE. The essential deming: leadership principles from the father of quality. New York: McGraw Hill Professional; 2012. ISBN 978-0-07-179021-5

Deming WE. Out of the crisis, reissue. Cambridge: MIT Press; 2018. ISBN 978-0-262-35003-7.

Deming WE, Massachusetts Institute of Technology. Center for Advanced Engineering Study. Quality, productivity, and competitive position. Cambridge: Massachusetts Institute of Technology; 1982. ISBN 978-0-911379-00-6.

West CP, Dyrbye LN, Sinsky C, et al. Resilience and burnout among physicians and the general US Working Population. JAMA Netw Open. 2020;3(7):e209385. https://doi.org/10.1001/jamanetworkopen.2020.9385.

Yates SW. Physician stress and burnout. Am J Med. 2020;133(2):160–4. https://www.aamc.org/system/files/c/2/472906-howmedicaleducationischanging.pdf.   (http://creativecommons.org/licenses/by-nc-nd/4.0/)

Chapter 9
Getting Paid by Insurance

9.1 Medicare

Medicare's low reimbursement does not cover the cost of provided care. The justification is that the health care entities could be more efficient, and that the shortfall is made up by the private insurance companies. In 2020, Medicare paid 84 cents for every dollar spent by hospitals, resulting in a $75.6 billion underpayment. The Medicare Payment Advisory Commission (MedPAC) found that in 2020, hospitals and health systems experienced a −8.5% margin on Medicare services in 2020. MedPAC projects that this margin will fall to −9% in 2022, and if COVID-19 relief funds are excluded, will decline even further.

Commercial plans want to use Medicare reimbursement as their benchmark, some already do. In South Florida, some commercial plans pay 60–80% of Medicare rates. This leads to hospital closures and reduced access to care. Medicare reimbursement is based on old data, and once in place, is not updated for a year. There is no allowance for inflation, increased staffing costs, and supply shortages. CMS' proposed inpatient payments for 2023 are lower than inpatient payments made in 2022. This highlights a flawed system considering rising inflation and the COVID-19 emergency.

Even setting a reimbursement amount does not guarantee that amount. The 2011 Budget Control Act imposed mandatory spending reductions, called "sequestration." This resulted in an arbitrary and automatic reduction of all Medicare payments. One-third of hospitals are operating in the red, and many rural hospitals are closing.

Decreasing reimbursement leads to poorer quality care. Would you work for less when the unfunded mandates, like EMR and the supposed "quality" control mandates, have increased your costs? Poorly trained and paid technicians do more of the exam, as do ancillary healthcare workers. This is a role for nurse practitioners, as most general office visits do not require a physician. Physicians are necessary for the more complicated cases. The EMR takes care of the supposed "quality control" measures as it automatically populates everything. Medicine is being killed, and patients suffer, but it's okay if it costs less, the corporations make a lot of money, and the public is deceived.

Suggested Reading

https://www.aha.org/fact-sheets/2020-01-07-fact-sheet-underpayment-medicare-and-medicaid.

https://www.brookings.edu/blog/usc-brookings-schaeffer-on-health-policy/2022/03/29/what-does-economy-wide-inflation-mean-for-the-prices-of-health-care-services-and-vice-versa/.

https://www.medpac.gov/wp-content/uploads/import_data/scrape_files/docs/default-source/reports/mar21_medpac_report_to_the_congress_sec.pdf.

Leung EH, et al. Opportunity cost of retinal detachment surgery vs office-based care. J Vitreoret Dis. 2022;6(4):278–83.

Chapter 10
What Are the Customer Experience Challenges in Healthcare?

Bolton's et al. paper, "Customer experience challenges: bringing together digital, physical and social realms," discusses the trends in digital, physical, and social areas and their impact upon the development of customized customer experiences. This experience is comprised of multiple interactions with a focus on the design and delivering of an optimized experience. The digital realm has changed customer's behavior and thereby their experience for content, expertise, and customized solutions in real time. The physical realm aided by technology enhances convenience and comfort. The social realm is the heart of the customer experience and is defined by the interactions among customers, employees, and others. That relationship increasingly involves technological interfaces. Word of mouth (WOM), smartphones, and social networks can be used to influence customers, both in a positive (convivial) and negative (crowding) direction.

Telemedicine without insurance reimbursement has been in use for the last decade. The COVID-19 pandemic and social distancing has now forced insurance companies to reimburse for the service and states to remove in-state licensing requirements for telemedicine providers. The "science-fiction" like promise of surgeons remotely operating on patients using robots has and will not be realized do to technological, equipment costs, liability, and reimbursement issues. The removal of "artificial" barriers will allow an

J. N. Weiss, *Physician Crisis*,
https://doi.org/10.1007/978-3-031-27979-9_10

increase in remote diagnosis with the development of therapeutic plans.

For-profit hospital systems have used telemedicine to their advantage. Services like radiology interpretation have been outsourced to other states and even other countries. And when the reading is incorrect, is the physician in another country libel for the mistake? If you're a plaintiff's attorney, you sue the closest physicians you can get your hands on, not someone 10,000 miles away in another country.

Clayton Christensen et al. "The Innovator's Prescription" speaks to the new era of "personalized medicine." This does not include the gratuitous use of robots as a marketing tool without true value. North Broward Hospital in Pompano Beach, Florida, (where I used to work) purchased several robots that would bring medications to the wards. Adding a new technological tool to an old infrastructure did not allow integration, the robot became a "toy," and was eventually discarded.

Likewise, the promise of the interconnectivity of Electronic Medical Records (EMR) has not been realized. Software remains proprietary and unable to connect with other hospital systems and physician offices using different software platforms. EMR use has resulted in an increase in paper utilization as what was previously contained in a one-page paper report now takes seven printed pages in an EMR report. The use of the EMR systems has dramatically increased physician discontent and burnout. Patients complain that the physician spends most of the examination time looking at a computer monitor and not at the patient. It is doubtful that EMR use has enhanced the quality of medical care but has greatly contributed to billing and insurance procedures. The loss of privacy and information sharing can also affect the development of the customer relationship.

Machines can display signs of empathy, without demonstrating or understanding the concept. The removal of technology, i.e., technological malfunction, may have disastrous consequences in the ability to retrieve medical records.

Critics have complained that while healthcare costs have increased, the customer experience has been poor.

The Merriam-Webster dictionary defines business competition "as the effort of two or more parties acting independently to secure the business of a third party by offering the most favorable terms." Competition stimulates firms to develop new products and services, which gives consumers greater selection, better products, and lower prices. However, as competition in healthcare has been stifled, customer service has generally become irrelevant.

A Certificate of Need (CON) is necessary for the construction, acquisition, creation, or expansion of a healthcare facility in an area to affirm that the plan is required to fulfill the needs of a community. A CON is necessary in 35 states and is issued by state health agencies to address concerns that the construction of excess hospital capacity would cause competitors in an oversaturated field to overcharge patients. Unfortunately, it grants monopoly status to existing hospitals by eliminating competition and creating the problem the CON was hoping to avoid.

When there is only one hospital in a given geographic area, good customer service is unnecessary. Both sick patients and ambulances go to the nearest hospital. Insurance also dictates to which hospital a patient may go. Hospitals are generally not "chosen." Patients who leave the hospital improved are happy. The patient condition, whether medical or surgical, takes precedence over whether the breakfast arrived on time. CONs are sold in bankruptcy as an asset, and the CON requirement is sometimes used by competitors to block the reopening of existing hospitals.

A 2011 study found that CONs "reduce the number of beds at the typical hospital by 12%, on average, and the number of hospitals per 100,000 persons by 48%. These reductions ultimately lead urban hospital CEOs in states with CON laws to extract economic rents of $91,000 annually." CONs have been blamed for the potential shortage of hospital beds during the COVID-19 pandemic.

As of 2020, there were 5198 community hospitals in the country, 2937 nongovernmental not-for-profit hospitals, 1296 for-profit hospitals, and 965 state and local government hospitals. The for-profit hospital sector is highly concentrated. Four health systems accounted for about 520 hospitals: Franklin, TN-based Community Hospital Systems (CHS); Nashville-based Hospital Corporation of America (HCA); Brentwood, TN-based LifePoint Health; and Dallas-based Tenet Healthcare Corporation.

Reductions in federal payments to hospitals will total $252.6 billion from 2010 through 2029, reflecting the cumulative impact of a series of legislative and regulatory actions. The American Hospital Association and the Federation of American Hospitals denounced the impact of the payment reductions on hospitals' financial health. Table 10.1 quantified the cumulative impact of payment reductions mandated in 12 legislative acts and numerous regulatory changes from CMS to reach the total dollar amount, which included federal payments for inpatient and outpatient acute care, freestanding inpatient rehabilitation, long-term care hospitals, inpatient psychiatric units, hospital-based rehabilitation, skilled nursing, and home health.

In addition to Medicare spending cuts, hospitals also face declining service volumes, rising costs, and a shrinking payer mix as more baby boomers shift from commercial insurers to Medicare.

The Dobson DaVanzo study analyzed the total impact of a series of budget acts mandating across-the-board cuts in federal spending, including an additional 2% reduction in Medicare payments due to sequestration; reductions in Medicare reimbursement to hospitals for bad debt; payment reductions in post-acute care, limitations on inflation-based payment increases in home health; adjustments to Medicare Severity diagnosis-related groups (MS-DRGs) payments; reductions in Medicaid disproportionate share payments; and other legislative changes.

In 2015, 40% of the highest Medicare-charging hospitals in the nation were in Florida and all were for-profit facilities.

TABLE 10.1 Drug approvals/biologic licenses

Act	Impact on Federal Payments to Hospitals
Sequestration	**$85.8**
Budget Control Act of 2011	$37.1
Bipartisan Budget Act of 2013	$10.3
Military Retiree COLA Restoration Bill of 2014	$5.6
Bipartisan Budget Act of 2015	$5.8
Bipartisan Budget Act of 2018	$12.7
Bipartisan Budget Act of 2019	$14.3
Payment of Medicare Bad Debt	**$5.7**
Middle Class Tax Relief and Job Creation Act of 2012	
Reduction in Post-Acute Care (PAC) Provider Payment Updates	**$7.3**
Medicare Access and CHIP Reauthorization Act of 2015	$6.8
Bipartisan Budget Act of 2018	$0.5
Hospital Documentation and Coding Adjustments	**$85.7**
American Taxpayer Relief Act of 2012	$10.95
Regulatory	$56.9
Medicare Access and CHIP Reauthorization Act of 2015	$16.8
21st Century Cures Act	$1.1
Off-Campus Provider Based Hospital Outpatient Departments	**$23.7**
Bipartisan Budget Act of 2015	$15.4
Regulatory	$8.3
Medicare Payments for Long Term Care Hospitals	**$8.1**
Bipartisan Budget Act of 2013	$7.8
Protecting Access to Medicare Act 2014	-$0.1
Bipartisan Budget Act 2018	$0.1
Regulatory	$0.3
Clarification of 3-Day Payment Window	**$4.2**
American Jobs and Closing Tax Loopholes Act of 2010	
Hospital Transfer Policy Expanded to Hospice	**$6.2**
Bipartisan Budget Act of 2018	
Federal Medicaid DSH Allotment Reductions [1]	**$25.9**
Multiple pieces of legislation	
Total Federal Reductions to Hospitals	**$252.6**

1/ The Medicaid DSH reduction factors in only the additional cut resulting from the legislative delays, for the period 2020 through 2025.
Source: Dobson | DaVanzo estimates – sources and methodology described above. Totals may not add due to rounding.

The analysis found that 49 of the 50 top Medicare charges are from for-profit facilities and half are owned by the for-profit hospital chain Community Health Systems. Twenty-eight percent of the hospitals are owned by the Hospital Corporation of America (HCA). The costs reports showed that the highest charging facilities had a markup of about ten times the Medicare allowable costs compared with a national average of 3.4 and a mode of 2.4.

In order to supposedly assess patient satisfaction, Medicare developed "The Hospital Consumer Assessment of Healthcare Providers and Systems" survey (HCAHPS). At discharge from the hospital, patients are asked 32 questions pertaining to their hospital stay. The resultant score determines whether the hospital gains or loses 2.0% of their Medicare payments. (With Medicare sequestration extended to 2030, the most funds a hospital may gain is 1.6%, not 2%.)

3553 U.S. hospitals received quality reviews of from 1 to 5 stars. 101 hospitals received the lowest ranking of one star (2.8%); 582 received two stars (16.4%); 1414 received three stars (39.8%); 1205 received four stars (33.9%); and 251 received the highest ranking of five stars (7.1%).

The summary rating includes an average of hospitals' performance on each of the 11 publicly reported measures from the Hospital Consumer Assessment of Healthcare Providers and Systems survey. The HCAHPS survey evaluates patients' experiences at the facilities.

The survey asks patients about factors such as the responsiveness of hospital staff to their needs, the quality of care transitions, and how well information about medications is communicated. It also asks about cleanliness and quietness of the facility and whether or not the patient would recommend it to others. The surveys are provided to a random sampling of patients within 2 days after they have been discharged from a hospital and must be completed within 42 days.

The average U.S. hospital score is 3–4 stars. Northwest Medical Center (HCA), Cleveland Clinic and Broward General Medical Center (North Broward Hospital District), all in Broward County, Florida, each earned 2 stars. North Broward Medical Center, also part of the North Broward Hospital District, earned 1 star. West Boca Medical Center and Delray Medical Center, both Tenet hospitals in Palm Beach County, earned 2 stars. All hospitals are geographically separated without local competition.

Northwest Medical Center, owned by HCA, consistently scores 1–2 stars, but is among the most profitable in the HCA group. Management receives bonuses for profitability.

Experienced personnel are terminated and replaced with new hires with little experience, patient waiting times are long, there is inadequate staffing, and employee morale is poor. The Medicare incentive is minimal, compared to the profit they are making.

The Memorial Hospital System (South Broward Hospital District) earned 4 stars. This is a public system that has had a top-level management team and has had quality appointed commissioners with healthcare experience for many years.

Unfortunately, the North Broward Hospital System has continually been plagued with self-dealing and dishonesty, culminating in multiple federal investigations and fines, firing of administrators and commissioners, and the suicide of a past CEO. The past Governor has used appointments to this Board as a gift to his loyal supporters. Money is wasted on unused and unnecessary equipment and sweetheart deals to friends.

Mayo Clinic in Jacksonville received 5 stars. The Mayo Clinic does not participate with Medicare, and only accepts in-state Medicaid, unlike the Cleveland Clinic which accepts all insurances. Not accepting the low Medicare reimbursement and not complying with their onerous regulations is a separating equilibrium between Mayo Clinic (5 stars) and Cleveland Clinic (2 stars). Reimbursement drives customer service and quality.

Chronic under-reimbursement of for-profit hospitals has led to the business decision to ignore customer service and focus on cost cutting, savings, and profit. Political influence and oversight by political appointees without healthcare experience resulted in poor customer service at the non-profit public North Broward Hospital district, whereas proper management with ethical controls resulted in good customer service at the non-profit public South Broward Hospital district. Cleveland Clinic, a non-profit private hospital accepts all insurance and consequently made the business decision to cut costs and customer service. Mayo Clinic, a non-profit private hospital system, does not accept low paying plans, including Medicare, and as a result is able to strengthen their brand with excellent customer service.

Suggested Reading

Boehm E. America doesn't have enough hospital beds to fight the coronavirus. Protectionist health care regulations are one reason why. 2020. Reason.com 2020-03-13. Accessed 24 May 2020.

Bolton RN, McColl-Kennedy JR, Cheung L, Gallan A, et al. Customer experience challenges: bringing together digital, physical and social realms. J Serv Manag. 2018;29(5):776–806.

Brown SW, Nelson AM, Bronkesh SJ, Wood SD. Quality service for practice success. Maryland: Aspen Publication; 1993.

Christensen CM, Grossman JH, Hwang J. The innovator's prescription: a disruptive solution for health care. New York: McGraw-Hill; 2009.

Eichmann TL, Santerre RE. Do hospital chief executive officers extract rents from certificate of need laws? J Health Care Finance. 2011;37(4):1–14.

Hall MF. Looking to improve financial results? Start by listening to patients. Healthc Financ Manage. 2008;62:76.

Hasin MAA, Seeluangsawat R, Shareef MA. Statistical measures of customer satisfaction for health care quality assurance: a case study. Int J Health Care Qual Assur. 2001;14(1):6–13.

Hein EC. Contemporary leadership behavior, selected readings. 5th ed. Philadelphia, NY: Lippincott; 1998.

Kohn LT, Committee on Quality of Health Care in America, IOM. Crossing the quality chasm: a new health system for the twenty-first century. Washington, DC: National Academy Press; 2001. p. 39–40.

Luecke RW, Rosselli VR, Moss JM. The economic ramifications of "client" dissatisfaction. Group Pract J. 1991:8–18.

McHugh MD, Kutney-Lee A, Cimiotti JP, Sloane DM, Aiken LH. Nurses' widespread job dissatisfaction, burnout, & frustration with health benefits signal problems for patient care. Health Aff (Millwood). 2011;30(2):202–10. J.D. Power and associates national hospital service performance study: (2020) https://www.hcahpsonline.org (/en/) Centers for Medicare & Medicaid Services, Baltimore, MD.

Naidu A. Factors affecting patient satisfaction and healthcare quality. Int J Health Care Qual Assur. 2009;22(4):366–81.

Ohlhausen MK. Certificate of need laws: a prescription for higher costs. Antitrust. 2015;30(1):50–4.

Poulas GA, Brodell RT, Mostow EN. Improving quality and patient satisfaction in dermatology office practice. Arch Dermatol. 2008;144:263–5.

Raposo ML, Alves HM, Duarte PA. Dimensions of service quality and satisfaction in healthcare: a patient's satisfaction index. Serv Bus. 2009;3:85–100.

Renzi C, Abeni D, Picardi A, et al. Factors associated with patient satisfaction with care among dermatological outpatients. Br J Dermatol. 2001;145:617–3.

Rice C. "5 ways to raise HCAHPS scores via staff engagement." Health Leaders Media Insider, November 2014.

Tabbish S. Hospital and health services administration principles and practice. Oxford: Oxford University Press; 2001. p. 699.

Voluntary Hospitals of America. Special report: quality care. Market Monitor. 1988:11.

Wendy L, Scott G. Service quality improvement: the customer satisfaction strategy for health care. American Hospital Pub; 1994.

Chapter 11
Drug Pricing

When pharmaceuticals are too expensive for the average person to afford, they either don't purchase them or use a lower dose so they will last longer. As a consequence, patients will suffer and will require more physician visits, which, due to insurance, may be free, or less expensive than the cost of the medication. It is a vicious cycle. Obviously, when Americans pay the highest drug prices in the world, and the same drug is available, frequently from the same manufacturer at a much lower price in another country, the system is broken. But there is too much money involved for it to be fixed in a sensible manner that benefits consumers. The government may subsidize patchwork improvements but what is needed is a complete overhaul and price controls.

The annual cost of wasteful spending from pharmaceutical pricing failure is estimated at approximately $230–$240 billion. New high-cost specialty drugs, i.e. cancer, will exceed 50% of pharmaceutical spending. Strategies to reduce drug costs include importation from lower cost countries, reforming price transparency, and competition.

How are prescription drug prices determined? Pharmaceutical companies make up one of the largest lobbying groups in congress. The American Medical Association (AMA) determined that many drug prices exceed the costs of research and development (R&D), or there may not be

© The Author(s), under exclusive license to Springer Nature
Switzerland AG 2023
J. N. Weiss, *Physician Crisis*,
https://doi.org/10.1007/978-3-031-27979-9_11

any R&D costs if the company purchases an existing drug. There is no transparency.

Pharmacy Benefit Managers work for health insurance companies to negotiate drug prices as well as rebates to the insurance company which are unseen by the consumer. The health insurance company may be rewarded by increasing the utilization of a particular drug on their formulary. Health Insurance Companies are allowed to negotiate as a block with drug companies but this has not occurred. German health insurance plans recently negotiated with pharmaceutical companies as a group and lowered overall German drug prices.

Pharmaceutical companies also establish patient advocacy groups, who on the surface, appear to be unbiased, but reflect the interests of the supporting drug companies. In addition, as the major financial supporters of Professional Physician Academies, the leaders of those organizations, whether instructed to do so, unconsciously, or to curry favor with the company in order to get a consulting contract, or a job, may reflect and protect the companies interests over those of their own members and intentionally stifle innovation hopefully to win praise from their financial "masters."

Business decisions are governed by money. Academic decisions are governed by money and ego. Human nature has not changed over a thousand years. When new research is quashed, the innovator criticized and expelled from mainstream medicine, it is to protect self-interest. This is in effect a monopoly that is hurting patients. Unfortunately, the legal system is geared to who has the best attorney's and the most money. Justice may be blind, but it is not deaf, and a judge doesn't have to expend any time or energy to support the larger entity. A single physician cannot fight a large professional academy or corporate interest. They have lawyers on retainer and you don't. You can't win, even if you are right.

The system is filled with lies. In a June 2019 report, the Council of Economic Advisers credited the Trump Administration's deregulation efforts with reducing healthcare prices. They also claim these efforts have enhanced "choice and price competition in the biopharmaceutical markets." These statements are not true. The observed reduction in pharmaceutical prices has been driven by the routine expiration of patents, which just so happened to occur for a few top selling pharmaceuticals, and the subsequent availability of generic substitutes. The moderate increase in the number of FDA approvals has not resulted in a reduction in pharmaceutical prices.

The Council of Economic Advisers (CEA) (2019a, b) also credited the Trump Administration's policies of deregulation in reducing healthcare prices. In particular, the CEA cited an 11% reduction in the trend price of prescription drugs as of May 2019. It attributed the decline to the 2017 Drug Competition Action Plan and the 2018 Strategic Policy Roadmap. These regulations, the CEA claimed, have enhanced "choice and price competition in the biopharmaceutical markets" and led the FDA to approve "a record number of generic and new brand name drugs."

Did the Trump Administration's policies truly affect the trend of reducing pharmaceutical prices? Did these policies have the rule of law, or did they just provide industry guidance? Or were there other factors in reducing the trend of price increases, such as the patent expiration of the most expensive drugs with the subsequent appearance of lower cost biosimilars and discounting?

The CEA credited two policies with reducing prescription drug prices: the 2017 Drug Competition Action Plan and the 2018 Strategic Policy Roadmap. Before considering the effects of these, it is worth reviewing precisely what, if anything, these policies have changed.

The 2017, FDA Drug Competition Action Plan focused on three key areas. The intention was to improve generic drug development and approval, improve regulatory clarity, and to close the loopholes that allow "brand-name" drug companies to delay generic drug competition. Unfortunately, the result was the publishing of draft guidance, updates, manuals, press releases and holding public meetings without any meaningful regulatory change.

In a January 2018 address, FDA Commissioner Scott Gottlieb, MD, described the "Healthy Innovation, Safer Families: FDA's 2018 Strategic Policy Roadmap." He identified four areas of focus for the FDA:

1. Reduce the burden of addiction crises that are threatening American families.
2. Leverage innovation and competition to improve healthcare, broaden access, and advance public health goals.
3. Empower consumers to make better and more informed decisions about their diets and health and expand the opportunities to use nutrition to reduce morbidity and mortality from disease.
4. Strengthen FDA's scientific workforce and its tools for efficient risk management.

No direct mention was made of reducing pharmaceutical costs or increasing the supply of generic drugs. Only the second goal would seem to deal with pharmaceutical costs. Unfortunately, once again, only draft guidance without any regulatory change was provided. The FDA offered to "streamline" generic drug development, but only "after all of the blocking patent and exclusivity periods have lapsed on branded medicine." Other nonsignificant changes in FDA regulations were also promoted.

Despite voicing the desire to reduce drug prices, President Trump and the Republican Party have consistently resisted efforts to do so. In 2019, the U.S. House of Representatives passed the Grassley-Wyden bill which would force drug makers to negotiate prices with Medicare. The bill stalled in the Senate and was opposed by the White House.

President Trump announced possible Executive Action where the cost of certain Medicare Part B drugs would be tied to the International Price Index. To support his effort, a recent White House study reiterated that "drug prices are suppressed overseas" and that "foreign governments are taking unfair advantage of American drug company research and U.S. consumers." Non-U.S. drug prices are frequently set by government run health care systems and are lower than U.S. prices. Unfortunately, this would utilize a socialist pricing model, which the President has consistently railed against.

The President has also recommended importation of drugs from Canada. However, both the pharmaceutical industry and the Canadian government are strongly opposed to these proposals and nothing has transpired.

In December 2019, the House of Representatives passed The Elijah E. Cummings Lower Drug Costs Now Act, which would allow Medicare to negotiate the prices of 250 drugs per year; cap drug payments at 120% of the average price in six other countries; prohibit price increases beyond the inflation rate; allow private insurers to purchase drugs at Medicare's prices; and cap out-of-pocket spending by seniors at $2000 per year. However, Senator Majority Leader Mitch McConnell called this "socialist price controls" and refused to address the bill in the Senate.

Senators Grassley (R-IA) and Wyden (D-OR) have intro-duced bipartisan legislation that would penalize drug compa-nies if they raise prices faster than inflation. However, other Republican senators opposed this bill for "price setting."

Therefore, despite protestations to the contrary, President Trump and the Republican Party have ignored every oppor-tunity to engage with the Democratic Party in meaningful legislation that would have the potential to reduce pharma-ceutical costs.

But, is the CEA correct? Did President Trump's new regu-lations and initiatives enhanced "choice and price competi-tion in the biopharmaceutical markets" and have they stimulated the FDA to approve "a record number of generic and new brand name drugs?" Are drug prices lower? If the trend of drug pricing is declining and the government's claims are correct, are they the result of their policies or of other factors?

Robinson et al. studied a drug pricing program utilized by the Reta Trust health insurance program. Employees paid more out-of-pocket costs if they chose more expensive drugs in a therapeutic class. (Of note, for every $1 pharmaceutical companies spend on advertising, they reap $2 in sales. Advertising drives the use of particular drugs, many of only marginal benefit over existing lower cost alternatives.) The study found that immediately after implementation the patient's mean out-of-pocket spending for drugs increased by 10% for the first 2 years and then decreased over time. While there may be competition between drugs in a particular class, drugs are not equivalent, which may provide hardship for some patients. An average decline in out-of-pocket prices does not translate into a lower out-of-pocket cost for all.

When the Medicare Part D drug benefit plan began in 2006, six classes of drugs were termed "protective classes," meaning Medicare could not negotiate prices. Yarbrough determined that the "protective" class of drugs led to an increase of $112–$121 million per drug per year in US sales relative to unprotected drugs. The protected drugs include anticancer, antidepressant, antipsychotic, and anticonvulsant drugs.

The National Center for Biotechnology Information performed an analysis of World Health Organization essential medicines in the Medicare Part D program from 2011 to 2015. The main outcome measures were total and per beneficiary Medicare spending, total and per beneficiary out-of-pocket patient spending, cumulative beneficiary count, claim count, and per unit drug cost. Measures were inflation adjusted and reported in 2015 US dollars.

There are 265 WHO essential medicines. From 2011–2015, the annual spending increased from $11.9 billion in 2011 to $24.8 billion, an 116% increase. Patient's annual spending was $12.1 billion. Total annual out-of-pocket patient spending for this period increased from $2.0 billion to $2.9 billion (47% increase); annual per beneficiary spending increase 4%. Prescription count increase from 376.1 million to 498.9 million (33% increase) and beneficiary count grew from 95.9 million to 135.8 million (42% increase).

Fifty percent of the essential drugs (133) increased faster than the average inflation rate. Fifty-eight percent of total spending increase was largely attributed to the introduction of two expensive drugs to treat hepatitis C. Twenty-two percent of increased spending was related to increase in per unit cost of existing drugs.

Drug approvals have increased under the Trump Administration. From 2016 to 2019, there was a 13% increase in Drug Approvals and a 12% increase in Biologic License approvals as compared to the period, 2012–2015. (Table 11.1).

TABLE 11.1   Drug approvals/biologic licenses

	# of FDA drug approvals by year	# of biologic licenses by year
2019	48	22
2018	59[a]	18
2017	46	18
2016	22	9
2015	45	12
2014	41	19
2013	27	17
2012	39	11

	Total FDA drug approvals	Total biologic licenses
2016–2019 President Trump	175	67
2012–2015 President Obama	152	59

[a] 43/59 (73%) used a shorter, expedited approval mechanism

11.1   Have Prescription Prices Decreased Under the Trump Administration?

(Note—biosimilars are the generic equivalent of a biologic drug)

The report states that the new FDA initiatives resulted in "the July 2017 crash of the stock of at least one foreign generic drug maker" which was attributed to greater competition as a result of increased FDA drug approvals. A closer analysis reveals that the company was found guilty of a coordinated scheme to artificially maintain high prices for a generic antibiotic and a diabetes drug. The complaint alleged price collusion between six pharmaceutical firms. Prices did fall as a result of the lawsuit, but it was due to state, not federal action, nor a result of federal policy but the discovery and prosecution of illegal activity. In May 2019, the same company was one of 19 drug companies sued for price fixing in the United States by 44 states for inflating its prices, sometimes up to 1000%, in an illegal agreement among it and its competitors.

From 2007 to 2018, the inflation adjusted list price of pharmaceuticals (wholesale acquisition price) increased 159% and the inflation adjusted net price (price after discounts and rebates) increased 60% for 602 drugs. Sixty-two percent of the increase in list prices was offset by discounts. Drug companies offer discounts to offset list price increase, restrain competition, improve market share through better formulary placement and to increase the volume of sales. Patients do not receive discounts; the uninsured, those with high-deductible plans, or in the deductible portion of their policy, pay the list price. Coinsurance payments are based on a percentage of the list price.

In 2020, the price of nearly 500 drugs increased an average of 5.2%. Humira's price increased 7.4%, which was in addition to the 19.1% price increase for 2018 and 2019. The Institute for Clinical and Economic Review determined that data did justify the large increase in price.

11.2 Best-Selling Prescription Drugs by Worldwide Revenue Under President Trump

May 2019

1. Humira $19.9 billion Accounts for approximately 61% of AbbVie's total revenue. Net sales grew 7% in 2018. Despite biosimilars (outside US)—growth occurred due to increase in indications. NHS (Great Britain) #1 purchased drug—switch to biosimilars saved approximately $200 million. U.S. patent expired 2016, HOWEVER— AbbVie has filed more than 100 additional patents to stave off biosimilars and extend patent protection beyond 2030. U.S. PATENTS IN FORCE.

2. Eliquis $9.8 billion 32% growth in 2018 U.S. PATENT IN FORCE.

3. Revlimid $9.7 billion 18% year over year growth U.S. PATENT IN FORCE.

4. Keytruda $7.1 billion 47% growth in 2018 worldwide, Off patent 2018—US/Europe, 2032—Japan. Keytruda manufactured by Merck. Strong competition by Bristol-Meyers Squibb's Obdivo (biosimilar). (4/20). US PATENT EXPIRED.

5. Enbrel $7.1 billion 8% sales drop 2017–2018, lower cost— Not approved for as many uses as Humira. Patent expiration 2019, 2023, 2028, 2029. Biosimilar developed (lower price) (4/20). U.S. PATENT EXPIRED.

6. Herceptin $7 billion. Patent expired 2019. 4 biosimilars with lower price, 16% decline in sales. U.S. PATENT EXPIRED.

7. Avastin $6.9 billion 3% growth due to 12% international growth, especially China. Patent expired 2019 US, 2022 Europe, U.S. PATENT EXPIRED Biosimilar exists (4/20).

8. Eylea $6.7 billion International sales increased by 12% in 2018 compared to 2017. U.S. AND EUROPEAN PATENTS EXPIRED No biosimilar (4/20).

9. Opdivo $6.7 billion sales 37% increase in 2018 and 36% worldwide 2018. U.S. PATENT IN FORCE.
10. Xarelto $6.5 billion 5% growth 2018–2017 U.S. patent expires 2024. Declining revenue due to greater discounts. Many personal injury lawsuits (approximately 25,000).

11.3   Best-Selling Prescription Drugs by Worldwide Revenue Under President Obama

December 2015

1. Humira Sales $14.0 Billion (Change from 2014 $1.47)
   #1 selling drug in 2019.
2. Harvoni Sales $13.9 Billion (Change from 2014 $11.7)
   Not top 10 selling drug in 2019.
   Patent expiring 2030.
3. Enbrel sales $8.7 billion (change from 2014 $4.0) #5 selling drug in 2019.
4. Remicade sales $8.4 billion (change from 2014 $1.5).
   Not top 10 selling drug in 2019.
   Patent expired 2017.
5. Rituxan Sales $7.1 Billion (Change from 2014 $1.5)
   Not top 10 selling drug in 2019.
   Patent expired 2018.
6. Lantus Sales $7.0 Billion (Change from 2014 $0.51)
   Not top 10 selling drug in 2019.
   Patent expiring 2028.
7. Avastin Sales $6.8 Billion (Change from 2014 $0.27)
   #7 top selling drug in 2019.
8. Herceptin Sales $6.6 Billion (Change from 2014 $0.27)
   #6 top selling drug in 2019.
9. Revlimid Sales $5.8 Billion (Change from 2014 $0.8)
   #3 top selling drug in 2019.
10. Sovaldi Sales $5.3 Billion (Change from 2014 $5.0)
    Not top 10 selling drug in 2019.
    Patent expiring 2034.

Five of the top selling drugs in 2015 were also the top selling drugs in 2019. Humira remained the #1 top selling drug in both groups, Enbrel dropped from #3 to #5, Avastin remained at #7 in both groups, Herceptin went from #8 (2015) to #6 (2019), and Revlimid from #9 (2015) to #3 (2019).

In 2015, under President Obama, all of the top 10 selling drugs were patent protected, there were no generics or biosimilars. Two of the top 10 selling drugs in 2015 lost patent protection in 2017 and 2018 and were no longer top selling drugs in 2019.

In 2019, of the 10 best-selling prescription drugs by revenue, 5 patents expired from 2018 to 2019 and 4 lower cost biosimilars now exist. One patented drug, Xarelto, has been forced to provide greater discounts. Off patent drugs without a biosimilar may be substantially discounted or subject to large rebates to discourage companies from producing biosimilars. Rebates are not subject to public scrutiny, nor reflected in wholesale prices. Therefore, the decrease in drug prices for these particular drugs was not the result of any Trump administration policies.

Drug prices have not decreased, but have increased under the Trump administration. The lower price of some pharmaceuticals is due to the loss of patent protection, generic formulations, and the actions of states in pursuing legal action against generic drug makers.

Note:

In 2022, President Biden was successful in signing the Inflation Reduction Act. Beginning in 2026, Medicare will have the ability to negotiate drug prices with pharmaceutical manufacturers for a select number of high-cost drugs. The program will reduce prices for selected drugs by 25–65%. Medicare will reimburse pharmacies thereby altering the "buy and bill" system through which pharmacies and providers presently purchase.

Suggested Reading

Barba V. Prices of nearly 500 drugs increased in 2020. Pharma Technologist.com. 1/8/20. 2020. https://www.in-pharmatechbnologist.com/Article/2020/01/08/Drugmakers-announce-drug-prices-increases-for-2020.

Chernow ME. Private sector strategies to address high drug prices and the promise of reference pricing programs. JAMA Netw Open. 2020;3(2):e1920599. https://doi.org/10.1001/jamanetworkopen.2019.20599.

Deb C, Curfman G. Relentless prescription drug price increases. JAMA. 2020;323(9):826–8.

FDA. Novel drug approvals for 2016. 2017. https://www.fda.gov/drugs/new-drugs-fda-cders-new-molecular-entities-and-new-therapeutic-biological-products/novel-drug-approvals-2016.

FDA. Healthy innovation, safer families: FDA's 2018 strategic policy roadmap. 2018a. https//www.fda.gov/about-fda/reports/healthy-innovation-safer-families-fdas-2018-strategic-policy-roadmap.

FDA. Novel drug approvals for 2017. 2018b. https://www.fda.gov/drugs/new-drugs-fda-cders-new-molecular-entities-and-new-therapeutic-biological-products/novel-drug-approvals-2017.

FDA. Novel drug approvals for 2018. 2019a. https://www.fda.gov/drugs/new-drugs-fda-cders-new-molecular-entities-and-new-therapeutic-biological-products/novel-drug-approvals-2018.

FDA. Advancing health through innovation: 2018 new drug therapy approvals. Report-2018 impact innovation predictability access. FDA's Center for Drug Evaluation and Research, January 2019. 2019b.

FDA. Novel drug approvals for 2019. 2020. https://www.fda.gov/drugs/new-drugs-fda-cders-new-molecular-entities-and-new-therapeutic-biological-products/novel-drug-approvals-2019.

FDA. Novel drug approvals for 2020. 2021. https://www.fda.gov/drugs/new-drugs-fda-cders-new-molecular-entities-and-new-therapeutic-biological-products/novel-drug-approvals-2020.

FDA. FDA drug competition action plan. 2022. https://www.fda.gov/drugs/guidance-compliance-regulatory-information/fda-drug-competition-action-plan.

Hernandez I, Good CB, Cutler DM, et al. The contribution of new product entry versus existing product inflation in the rising costs of drugs. Health Aff. 2019;38(1):76–83. https://doi.org/10.1377/hlthaff.2018.05147.

Hernandez I, San-Juan-Rodriguez GC, Gellad WF. Changes in list prices, net prices, and discounts for branded drugs in the US, 2007–2018. JAMA. 2020;323(9):854–62. https://doi.org/10.1001/jama.2020.1012.

Hwang TJ, Dusetzina SB, Feng J, et al. Price increases of protected-class drug in medicare part D, relative to inflation, 2012-2017. JAMA. 2019;322(3):267–9. https://doi.org/10.1001/jama.2019.7521.

Li DG, Najafzadeh M, Kesselheim AS, Mostaghimi A. Spending on World Health Organization essential medicines in medicare part D, 201–15: retrospective cost analysis. BMJ. 2019;366:l4257. https://www.ncbi.nlm.nih.gov/pubmed/31315833

Munos BH, Orloff JJ. Disruptive innovation and transformation of the drug discovery and development enterprise. National Academy of Medicine, Washington, DC. 2016. https://nam.edu/wp-content/uploads/2016/07.

Pharmaceutical Technology. The top selling prescription drugs by revenue. 2019. https://www.pharmaceutical-technology.com/features/top-selling-prescription-drugs.

Rind DM, Agboola F, Kumar VM, et al. Unsupported price increase report: 2019 assessment. Boston, MA: Institute for Clinical and Economic Review; 2019. https://icer-review.org/wp-content/uploads/2019/01/ICER_UPI_Final_Report_and_Assessment_110619.pdf

Robinson JC, Panteli D. Single-payer drug pricing in a multipayer health system: does Germany offer a model for the US? Health Affairs, 2019. 3/22/19 10.1377/hblog20190318.475434.

Robinson JC, Whaley C, Brown TT, Dhruva SS. Physician and patient adjustment to reference pricing for drugs. JAMA Netw Open. 2020;3(2):e1920544. https://doi.org/10.1001/jamanetworkopen.2019.20544.

Rowland C. Investigation of generic cartel expands to 300 drugs. Washington Post 12/9/18 Business (Economy). 2018.

Rubin R. Rebates–the little known factor behind increasing drug list prices. JAMA. 2020;323(9):812–3.

Shrank WH, Rogstad TL, Parekh N. Waste in the US health care system: estimated costs and potential for savings. JAMA. 2019;322(15):1501–9. https://doi.org/10.1001/jama.2019.13978.

Thomas K. News of charges in price-fixing inquiry sends pharmaceuticals tumbling. New York Times. 11/4/16 B(5). 2016.

US Food and Drug Administration. Orange book: approved drug products with therapeutic equivalence evaluations. 2020. https://www.accessdatafda.gov/scripts/cder/ob/patent_info.cfm?Product_No=002&Appl_No=021752&Appl_type=N. Accessed 2 Nov 2020.

White House. The economic effects of Federal Deregulation since January 2017: an interim report. The Council of Economic Advisers, June 2019. 2019a.

White House. Measuring prescription drug prices: a primer on the CPI prescription drug index. The Council of Economic Advisers, October 2019. 2019b.

Wineinger NE, Zhang Y, Topol EJ. Trends in prices of popular brand-name prescription drugs in the United States. JAMA Netw Open. 2019;2(5):e194791. https://doi.org/10.1001/jamanetworkopen.2019.4791.

Wingrove J. Trump eyes drug-price cuts after his health-care record is attacked. 2020. https://www.bloomberg.com/news/articles/2020-02-10.

Wouters OJ. Lobbying expenditures and campaign contributions by the pharmaceutical and health product industry in the United States. 1999-2018. JAMA Intern Med. 180:688. https://doi.org/10.1001/jamainternmed.2020.0146.

Yarbrough CR. How protected classes in Medicare part D influence U.S. drug sales, utilization, and price. Health Econ. 2020;29:608. https://doi.org/10.1002/hec.4006.

Chapter 12
"Malpractice"

A bad outcome is not necessarily malpractice nor negligence. The patient doesn't always "do well," like they generally do at the end of a television show. Treatments and surgery are not always successful, patients may continue to get sicker, depending on their medical condition, and die. Not all surgery is "successful." Medical care has risks.

The tort liability system is intended to serve three functions: compensate patients who sustain injury from negligence, provide corrective justice, and deter negligence. The threat of being sued is intended to deter a physician from negligently injuring patients. But this is not how it is working out. Patients sue for bad results, not due to negligence, and the high legal expenses in defending against claims force a settlement, whether it is justified or not, even more so since juries are uneducated to complex medical problems and are sympathetic to claimants.

Frivolous lawsuits are filed because the plaintiff's attorney knows that the insurance company will settle, to avoid the expenses of defending against the claim and possibly going to court. Depending on the settlement amount, the physician is reported to the National Practitioner Data Bank, and the settlement follows him or her around on every hospital, surgery center and insurance application, and state websites for years.

© The Author(s), under exclusive license to Springer Nature Switzerland AG 2023
J. N. Weiss, *Physician Crisis*,
https://doi.org/10.1007/978-3-031-27979-9_12

If one physician in a group of physicians treating the patient who is suing has insurance, that is the one who will be sued, whether or not that physician had any significant role in the patient's outcome. Also unfortunately, the race and ethnicity of the patient and the physician, depending on the population of the jurisdiction and the jury makeup, may also force the insurance company to settle. It becomes a money grab without a basis in right or wrong.

The physicians' reputation may be ruined, he/she must spend time and money fighting a frivolous claim, there is an emotional toll, all while the plaintiff's attorney and patient have nothing to lose. In other countries, if the judge rules the case frivolous, the plaintiff's attorney must pay the physician's legal fees. In the U.S., where trial attorney's control state legislatures, nothing like that is possible. Doctors become more cautious and take less risk, even when taking a risk is in the patient's best interest and only hope. Physicians, airline pilots, and police are held to the highest standards in the world. Everyone else, can just say "sorry," with little repercussion.

But does the risk of a lawsuit affect patient outcome? In a review of 37 studies,

28 examined hospital care, and 16 obstetrical care. Zero of the 7 studies that examined hospital readmissions and avoidable initial hospitalizations found an association between outcomes and the risk of liability. Of the 12 studies of other hospital measures, including quality of care and patient satisfactions, 7 found no association between outcomes and liability risk, 5 studies identified significant associations in some analyses.

In the obstetrical care studies, 9 found no significant association between outcomes and liability risk and 7 found a limited association. There were 20 studies of patient mortality, 15 found no evidence of an association of outcomes with liability risk, and 5 found limited evidence.

The evidence indicates that liability risk is not associated with improved quality of care. The defenders of the present system realize that though patients may not be compensated for their injury, nor provides a corrective justice, it does provide deterrence. But is this true?

Deterrence leads to making safe decisions, which may not benefit the patient when a riskier approach is necessary for a better outcome. Taking it a step further, the result is defensive medicine which provides minimal or no clinical benefit at increased cost, other than protecting the physician from liability. An unfortunate biproduct of the malpractice climate is that errors are swept under the rug and the problems are not solved and quality is not improved, because the physician fears litigation.

How Would a Deterrence Effect Work?
1. Malpractice awards are financial and affect credentialing by hospitals and insurance companies. Having malpractice insurance puts a target on your back. More and more physicians are "going bare," and not purchasing malpractice insurance. They are responsible for any legal fees, whether defending a valid or frivolous case. They are also responsible to pay any award. However, physicians may purchase "legal insurance," which covers the costs of attorney's fees up to a preset amount, but does not pay judgments.
2. Plaintiff's lawyers prefer suing the physician with the "deep pocket," that is, the one that has malpractice insurance, so they are guaranteed payment, and may settle the case without the physician's approval. And once the insurance company settles a case, the physician is frequently dropped from insurance. Any subsequent policy will be at a much greater cost, if the physician can even obtain one.
3. There is a psychological stress of litigation. This manifests itself in anger, shame, and second guessing by the physician.
4. The physicians practice may be limited by the hospital who views the lawsuit as a deviation from standard of care, whether it is or not.

The nature of medicine is that physicians want to do a good job and help the patient. That's why they became a physician. But like everyone else, they are human. Having the "Sword of Damocles" hanging over your head doesn't make you do better. Mistakes are made. Unfortunately, unlike cockpit errors in airplanes, physicians can't talk or implement fixes without the risk of a lawsuit and investigation by the Board of Medicine, a supposedly apolitical body that may not be friendly to the physician.

Most studies find no association between malpractice liability risk and healthcare quality and outcomes.

These are the five states with the lowest malpractice risk:

1. North Dakota—Noneconomic damages limited to $500,000. If noneconomic damages exceed $250,000, there is an additional review.
2. Wisconsin—Noneconomic damages of $750,000. Patient compensation fund pays for damages exceeding the cap.
3. Minnesota—Medical experts must confirm the merit of a claim—significant decrease in frivolous lawsuits.
4. Hawaii—$375,000 cap on noneconomic damage. Initial claims reviewed by a "Conciliation Panel."
5. North Carolina—Noneconomic damages capped at $500,000.

States with highest malpractice risk:

1. New Jersey
2. Louisiana
3. Pennsylvania
4. Florida
5. New York

Suggested Reading

Avraham R, Schanzenbach M. The impact of tort reform on intensity of treatment: evidence from heart patients. J Health Econ. 2015;39:273–88.

Baicker K, Chandra A. The effect of malpractice liability on the delivery of health care. Forum for Health Econ & Pol'y. 2005;8(1):841–52.

Baicker K, Fisher ES, Chandra A. Malpractice liability costs and the practice of medicine in the Medicare program. Health Aff (Millwood). 2007;26(3):841–52.

Balch CM, Oreskovich MR, Dyrbye LN, et al. Personal consequences of malpractice lawsuits on American surgeons. J Am Coll Surg. 2011;213(5):657–67.

Bartlett B. Legal epidemiology and the correlation of patient safety, deterrence, and defensive medicine. https://papers.ssrn.com/sol3/papers.cfm?abstract_id=2807689. 2017. Accessed June 4, 2019.

Bekelis K, Missios S, Wong K, MacKenzie TA. The practice of cranial neurosurgery and the malpractice liability environment in the United States. PLoS One. 2015;10(3):e0121191.

Bilimoria KY, Chung JW, Minami CA, et al. Relationship between state malpractice environment and quality of health care in the United States. Jt Comm J Qual Patient Saf. 2017;43(5):241–50.

Bilimoria KY, Sohn M-W, Chung JW, et al. Association between state medical malpractice environment and surgical quality and cost in the United States. Ann Surg. 2016;263(6):1126–32.

Black BS, Wagner AR, Zabinski Z. The association between patient safety indicators and medical malpractice risk: evidence from Florida and Texas. Am J Health Econ. 2017;3(2):109–39.

Boothman RC, Blackwell AC, Campbell DA Jr, et al. A better approach to medical malpractice claims? The University of Michigan experience. J Health Life Sci Law. 2009;2(2):125–59.

Carlson J, Foster K, Black B, et al. Emergency physician practice changes after being named in a malpractice claim. Ann Emerg Med. 2019;1–15

Charles SC, Pyskoty CE, Nelson A. Physicians on trial--self-reported reactions to malpractice trials. West J Med 1988; 148(3): 358–360.

Currie J, MacLeod WB. First do no harm? Tort reform and birth outcomes. Q J Econ. 2008;123(2):795–830.

Dhankhar P, Khan MM. Threat of malpractice lawsuit, physician behavior and health outcomes: a re-evaluation of practice of "defensive medicine" in obstetric care. 2009.

Dhankhar P, Khan MM, Bagga S. Effect of medical malpractice on resource use and mortality of AMI patients. J Empir Leg Stud. 2007;4(1):163–83.

Donabedian A. The quality of care. How can it be assessed? JAMA. 1988;260(12):1743–8.

Dranove D, Ramanarayanan S, Watanabe Y. Delivering bad news: market responses to negligence. J Law Econ. 2012;55(1):1–25.

Dubay L, Kaestner R, Waidmann T. The impact of malpractice fears on cesarean section rates. J Health Econ. 1999;18(4):491–522.

Dubay L, Kaestner R, Waidmann T. Medical malpractice liability and its effect on prenatal care utilization and infant health. J Health Econ. 2001;20(4):591–611.

Entman SS, Glass CA, Hickson GB, et al. The relationship between malpractice claims history and subsequent obstetric care. JAMA. 1994;272(20):1588–91.

Frakes M. Defensive medicine and obstetric practices. J Empir Leg Stud. 2012;9(3):457–81.

Frakes M, Gruber J. Defensive medicine: evidence from military immunity. 2018. https://papers.ssrn.com/sol3/papers.cfm?abstract_id=3218097. Accessed June 4, 2019.

Frakes M, Jena AB. Does medical malpractice law improve health care quality? J Public Econ. 2016;143:142–58.

Grady MF. Better medicine causes more lawsuits, and new administrative courts will not solve the problem. Northwestern Univ Law Rev. 1992;86(4):1068–93.

Hyman DA, Black B, Zeiler K, Silver C, Sage WM. Do defendants pay what juries award? Post-verdict haircuts in Texas medical malpractice cases, 1988–2003. J Empir Leg Stud. 2007;4(1):3–68.

Iizuka T. Does higher malpractice pressure deter medical errors? J Law Econ. 2013;56:161–88.

Keeton WP, Dobbs DB, Keeton RE, Owen DC. Prosser and Keeton on the law of torts. fifth ed. St. Paul, Minn: West Group; 1984.

Kessler D, McClellan M. Do doctors practice defensive medicine? Q J Econ. 1996;111:353–90.

Kessler D, McClellan M. Malpractice law and health care reform: optimal liability policy in an era of managed care. J Public Econ. 2002;84(2):175–97.

Kim B. The impact of malpractice risk on the use of obstetrics procedures. J Leg Stud. 2007;36:S79–S119.

Klick J, Stratmann T. Medical malpractice reform and physicians in high-risk states. J Leg Stud. 2007;36(2):S121–42.

Kohn LT, Corrigan JM, Donaldson MS, editors. To err is human: building a safer health system. Washington, D.C.: National Academies Press; 2000.

Konety BR, Dhawan V, Allareddy V, Joslyn SA. Impact of malpractice caps on use and outcomes of radical cystectomy for bladder cancer: data from the surveillance, epidemiology, and end results program. J Urol. 2005;173(6):2085–9.

Konetzka RT, Park J, Ellis R, Abbo E. Malpractice litigation and nursing home quality of care. Health Serv Res. 2013;48(6 Pt 1):1920–38.

Lakdawalla DN, Seabury SA. The welfare effects of medical malpractice liability. Int Rev. Law Econ. 2012;32(4):356–69.

Leape LL. Error in medicine. JAMA. 1994;272(23):1851–7.

Malak N, Yang Y. A re-examination of the effects of tort reforms on obstetrical procedures and health outcomes. Econ Lett. 2019;184:108626.

McMichael B. The failure of "sorry": an empirical evaluation of apology laws, health care, and medical malpractice. Lewis & Clark Law Rev. 2018;22(4):11991281.

Mello MM, Brennan TA. Deterrence of medical errors: theory and evidence for malpractice reform. Tex Law Rev. 2002;80(7):1595–637.

Mello MM, Chandra A, Gawande AA, Studdert DM. National costs of the medical liability system. Health Aff (Millwood). 2010;29(9):1569–77.

Mello MM, Hemenway D. Medical malpractice as an epidemiological problem. Soc Sci Med. 2004;59(1):39–46.

Minami CA, Sheils CR, Pavey E, et al. Association between state medical malpractice environment and postoperative outcomes in the United States. J Am Coll Surg. 2017;224(3):310–318 e312.

Missios S, Bekelis K. Spine surgery and malpractice liability in the United States. Spine J. 2015;15(7):1602–8.

Moghtaderi A, Farmer S, Black B. Damage caps and defensive medicine: reexamination with patient-level data. J Empir Leg Stud. 2019;16(1):26–68.

Schwartz GT. Reality in the economic analysis of tort law: does tort law really deter? UCLA Law Rev. 1994;42(2):377–444.

Sedgwick P. Ecological studies: advantages and disadvantages. BMJ. 2014;348:g 2979.

Shepherd JM. Tort reforms' winners and losers: the competing effects of care and activity levels. UCLA Law Rev. 2008;55(4):905–77.

Sloan FA, Entman SS, Reilly BA, et al. Tort liability and obstetricians' care levels. Int Rev. Law Econ. 1997;17(2):245–60.

Sloan FA, Shadle JH. Is there empirical evidence for "defensive medicine"? A reassessment J Health Econ. 2009;28(2):481–91.

Sloan FA, Whetten-Goldstein K, Githens PB, Entman SS. Effects of the threat of medical malpractice litigation and other factors on birth outcomes. Med Care. 1995;33(7):700–14.

Stevenson DG, Spittal MJ, Studdert DM. Does litigation increase or decrease health care quality: a national study of negligence claims against nursing homes. Med Care. 2013;51(5):430–6.

Studdert DM, Mello MM. In from the cold? Law's evolving role in patient safety. DePaul Law Rev. 2019;68(2):421–58.

Studdert DM, Mello MM, Brennan TA. Medical malpractice. N Engl J Med. 2004;350(3):283–92.

Yang YT, Mello MM, Subramanian SV, Studdert DM. Relationship between malpractice litigation pressure and rates of cesarean section and vaginal birth after cesarean section. Med Care. 2009;47(2):234–42.

Yang YT, Studdert DM, Subramanian SV, Mello MM. Does tort law improve the health of newborns, or miscarry? A longitudinal analysis of the effect of liability pressure on birth outcomes. J Empir Leg Stud. 2012;9(2):217–45.

Zabinski Z, Black BS. The deterrent effect of tort law: evidence from medical malpractice reform. https://papers.ssrn.com/sol3/papers.cfm?abstract_id=2161362. 2018. Accessed June 4, 2019.

Chapter 13
Private Equity

The Journal of the American Medical Association (JAMA) reported that of the approximately 18,000 group medical practices (2013–2016), there were 355 private equity practice acquisitions. Anesthesiology and multispecialty groups made up 19.4, emergency medicine 12.1%, family practice 11.1%, and dermatology 9.9%. There was also an increase in the number of acquired cardiology, ophthalmology, radiology, and obstetrics/gynecology practices from 2015 to 2016. Most acquired practices were in the South (44%). The acquired practices had several sites and a large practice volume. Surgical specialties offer increased revenues through added services like, ambulatory surgery centers, imaging, and laboratory.

Physicians receive a buyout plus equity in the new company. Investors are looking to recoup their investment in 3–5 years with a three to five times return on investment. The private equity firm will expand markets, decrease costs, acquire additional practices to join the larger practice, and recruit additional physicians. However, equity-backed physician staffing and management companies have been implicated in sending "out of network" surprise bills to emergency room patients.

The potential advantages of selling to a private equity group are that physicians have an exit strategy, the nonmedical aspects of the practice are now handled by another entity,

© The Author(s), under exclusive license to Springer Nature Switzerland AG 2023
J. N. Weiss, *Physician Crisis*,
https://doi.org/10.1007/978-3-031-27979-9_13

increased efficiencies, the ability to negotiate insurance contracts with higher reimbursement, and to incorporate new technologies. The downside, depending on the company, is that the maximization of profit may affect practice quality and patient care.

Suggested Reading

Shryock T. Private equity in healthcare. Med Econ J. 2019;96(22)

Zhu JM, Hua LM, Polsky D. Private equity acquisitions of physician medical groups across specialties, 2013–2016. JAMA. 2020;323(7):663–5. https://doi.org/10.1001/jama.2019.21844.

Chapter 14
What Country Has the Best Healthcare in the World?

The World Health Organization ranked these 10 countries as having the best healthcare in the world:

1. France
2. Italy
3. San Marino
4. Andorra
5. Malta
6. Singapore
7. Spain
8. Oman
9. Austria
10. Japan

Let's look at healthcare in larger countries:

France—Universal coverage. The government refunds most out-of-pocket fees.

Germany—Mixed public-private system, funded by statutory contributions. Advanced medical technology.

United Kingdom—Universal, government run. Accessibility problems. More than 10% of population buys private insurance for faster access to healthcare system.

Australia—Rated excellent for health outcomes. Universal Medicare system has covered the cost of public hospital stays.

Switzerland—Mandatory private health insurance with government involvement.

© The Author(s), under exclusive license to Springer Nature Switzerland AG 2023
J. N. Weiss, *Physician Crisis*,
https://doi.org/10.1007/978-3-031-27979-9_14

The Netherlands—Adults required to purchase basic health insurance. Employer payments and taxes help finance healthcare.

Japan—The statutory health insurance system (SHIS) covers more than 98% of Japan's population, while a separate system for those in poverty picks up the rest, proving itself as one of the countries with best healthcare in the world.

Japan's statutory health insurance covers the vast majority of treatments, including mental health care, hospice care, and most dental care. The idea of general practice is a recent one—most healthcare happens in privately owned specialist clinics.

Many countries have a single-payer healthcare that is universal and funded by the government. The government removes all competition in the market to keep costs low and standardize benefits. The national health service controls what "in-network" providers can do and what they can charge. Funded by taxes, there are no out-of-pocket fees for patients or any cost sharing. This system is used by the UK, Russia, UAE, Spain, Hong Kong, and other countries.

Another healthcare system option is where employers and employees are responsible for funding their health insurance system through "sickness funds" created by payroll deductions. Providers and hospitals are generally private, though insurers are public. In some instances, there is a single insurer (France, Korea). Other countries, like Germany and the Czech Republic, have multiple competing insurers. It is also used by some employer-based healthcare plans in the U.S.

A third popular option is the national health insurance model that is driven by private providers, but the payments come from a government-run insurance program that every citizen pays into. Essentially, the national health insurance model is universal insurance that doesn't make a profit or deny claims. In this case, some citizens have private health insurance, some may receive subsidized public healthcare, while some are not insured at all. It is used in China and Japan among others.

The out-of-pocket model is the most common model in less-developed areas and countries where there aren't enough financial resources to create a medical system like the models above. Patients must pay for their procedures out of pocket. It is used by Congo, Ethiopia, and some other countries around the world.

14.1   United States Healthcare

The U.S. spends the most per capita on healthcare than any country in the world, yet scores poorly on health care measures including maternal mortality, preventable hospital admissions, and life expectancy. All with a relatively low satisfaction index.

14.1.1   U.S.

Financial Burden

1. Un/under insured
2. Hidden prices
3. Surprise billing by out of network physicians or laboratories
4. Access problems
5. Health insurance may be lost if lose employment.
6. Health insurers restrict care to save money. This leads to no care or a delay in care, more suffering, and to worse and more expensive health outcomes.

Mis-Investments in Healthcare

- The medical system is focused on treating, not preventing disease. Procedures are paid at a better rate than is cognitive care. In home respiratory care, speech therapy, or psychological care may be "covered" by insurance, but the payment level is so low, that these services are unavailable because the therapists refuse to participate in the insurance plans.

The Stifling of Innovation

I am a retinal specialist and was trained in the use of a scleral buckle (a piece of silicone is placed around the eye) and vitrectomy (the vitreous body within the eye is removed) in the treatment of retinal detachments. These are two distinct procedures that were paid for separately. Medicare reduced the amount they paid for vitrectomy and now "included" the placement of a scleral buckle in the lower payment. Since scleral buckle placement is time consuming and difficult, requiring specialized training, and vitrectomy is faster and easier to perform, surgeons stopped performing scleral buckles. Retinal reattachment rates suffered. A second vitrectomy may be necessary, but when performed with the postoperative period of 90 days from the first vitrectomy, payment is even further reduced. New retinal specialists are no longer taught how to perform scleral buckles which involve suturing to the eye. Since vitrectomy surgery does not involve suturing, the new doctors don't know how to suture the eye, which is a very useful and important technique, and necessary if the eye is ruptured. A scleral buckle is a very good operation. But when reimbursement is low, or zero, the time and expertise necessary to perform the surgery disappears. This is how the government and insurance companies "practice" medicine.

A recent study demonstrated that even the amount Medicare pays for vitrectomy does not cover the cost of the procedure. Ophthalmology which used to be a lucrative specialty has been ostracized to surgery centers, because hospitals aren't reimbursed enough to pay for their costs, yet alone, make a profit.

Now even famous eye hospitals are closing, their buildings converted to office space or condominiums. Of course, private insurance companies use Medicare's codes, they "include" the scleral buckle payment with the vitrectomy as well. It is analogous to including two entrees in one dinner charge. Since there is only one code, it is impossible to know how many, if any, scleral buckles are being performed today.

Telehealth was not reimbursed before the COVID 19 pandemic. Why? Because it was an extra expense that more patients could utilize. But it is reimbursed now, by necessity, and is a valuable tool in bringing medical care not only during a pandemic, but to people with poor access to care, such as the poor, and disabled.

Home-based treatments, may be cost-effective and preferred by patients, are rarely covered. Insurance companies are profit making businesses, not charitable organization with empathy. As the telehealth example illustrates, they have to be forced into expanding services and spending more money.

When a claim is denied, and the physician or patient resubmits, the insurance company will ask for more information, then even more information, then the patient or physician will receive a denial letter saying that the plan does not cover this therapy; which the insurance company knew from the very beginning, but were hoping that the patient or physician would get discouraged and go away.

Another insurance "out" is stating that a particular treatment or procedure is "experimental." What does "experimental" mean? That is not "standard of care." But when the standard of care is to do nothing, and the patient will die or lose their vision, and a procedure that has published 15 peer-reviewed papers demonstrating efficacy, but not every doctor is performing it, is denied, is this right? And how will something become "standard of care" if it isn't paid for? No one could do it for free? They may have legal justification for their actions, but not moral support. Legal doesn't mean justice. And this is the disconnect. Insurance companies, both government and private, and companies, do not have a soul. The patient must be their own advocate in the current U.S. healthcare system. These people are "not your friends," they don't really care about you, it's just business to them.

One insurance company insisted that the physician, not an office person, ask for the approval to perform a procedure. I was connected to someone who didn't know what an ophthal-mologist was, and thought that there were just "eye doctors." She questioned why someone who fit eyeglasses was asking for an authorization to fix a retinal detachment.

A one-eyed Canadian attorney presented to my office with a retinal detachment in his only eye. He had Ontario Canada insurance. His company refused authorization for me to perform surgery. They insisted he drive back to Canada for "free" surgery. I explained that he had lost the vision in his only eye, he could not drive a car. They said then he should fly home. I operated, fixed his eye, his vision returned, but I never received payment.

In another case, a Medicare patient with proliferative dia-betic retinopathy underwent laser photocoagulation treatment of the eye in Tampa, Florida. He was visiting his son near my office, 5 h from Tampa, when his eye began to bleed. He presented to my office and I wanted to add more laser treatment in order to stop the bleeding. Medicare refused to pay me. Since the physician in Tampa had per-formed the first treatment, any subsequent treatment within 90 days was "included" in the Medicare payment to the other physician. Medicare said that he should have returned to Tampa, 5 h away from my office. I performed the treatment and was never paid.

When simple and effective procedures are paid at a "too low" reimbursement level, physicians will perform more com-plicated and better reimbursed procedures. When tests are inadequately reimbursed, physicians will perform more tests. It is not only greed for the additional money, sometimes it is to stay in practice and survive.

There is a simple in-office procedure that can repair a reti-nal detachment. The gas that we placed into the eye was not FDA approved, cost $70 a cannister, and was in use by retinal surgeons for 20 years without incident. The canister stated "not for human use" but there was no alternative, and every-one used it. Years later a company obtained FDA approved, and though the gas was still made by the same company, and came in the exact same cannister, it now had an FDA approved label, and a new price tag of $1500. Then, Medicare reduced the reimbursement for its use despite the fact that the physicians had to pay more for the gas. So retinal specialists now perform a more complicated and better reimbursed procedure instead. Every action has a reaction.

People travel, may go to a multiple of physicians, and switch physicians due to a myriad of reasons, including a change in health plans; medical care may be fragmented. This can lead to duplication of care, with poor coordination and higher costs.

A medication prescribed by one physician will rarely be discontinued by another physician and may be continued indefinitely, possible interacting with later prescribed medicines. Physicians don't have the time to exhaustively review a patient's medical history, more so because of the huge volume of EMR data. The promise of EMR interconnectivity has not been realized, and physicians are loath to share notes. Most record releases that my office sent out were rarely complied with, though it is the law to do so. Doctors repeat blood tests performed elsewhere because they don't have access to the prior results, are concerned with liability, or just want the additional income.

All you need is for a majority of people to be satisfied with their health care. They don't have to be happy or delighted, just satisfied, to keep the unhappy or excluded people from fighting to change the system.

Suggested Reading

Mirror, mirror 2021: reflecting poorly. https://www.commonwealthfund.org. Accessed 4 Jan 2022.
https://worldpopulationreview.com/country-rankings/best-healthcare-in-the-world. Accessed 4 Mar 2022.

Chapter 15
The Health Insurance Portability and Accountability Act (HIPAA)

The Health Insurance Portability and Accountability Act (HIPAA) was a good idea. But it has gotten out of control. All medical professionals are frightened of either a real or perceived violation that will get them in trouble. So, under the guise of HIPPA, no one tells anyone anything. Why risk the liability in a flawed legal system which isn't based upon common sense, but on who has the better lawyer and the power to win money?

I am continuously receiving privacy policies. Do you ever read them? Wasted effort. Yet the policy allows the company to release certain information without your additional consent. But physician, billing offices, and insurance companies are frightened and frequently won't release any information, even when the information if released will benefit the patient.

When my mother was very ill, and incapacitated, she received a bill from the hospital. It was a standard bill, without any itemization or note. I called the billing office and asked what it was for. They refused to tell me. I replied that I wanted to pay the bill but before I pay it, want to know what it is for. They refused to tell me. They wanted to speak to my mother, who unfortunately could no longer speak. We went around and around in circles and nothing was accomplished. The bill was never paid.

Refusing to release important medical information jeopardizes patient care. It also inhibits learning, which also results

© The Author(s), under exclusive license to Springer Nature Switzerland AG 2023
J. N. Weiss, *Physician Crisis*,
https://doi.org/10.1007/978-3-031-27979-9_15

in a decrease in the quality of medical care. There is a culture of paranoia.

And when family members call wanting to know how their relative is doing? Sometimes, family members will tell the doctor not to speak to a certain member. Or what happens when it is a blended family, or there was a divorce? The physician does not want to be cruel, but doesn't want to be brought up on charges of a HIPPA violation.

Hospital and office rooms needed to be redesigned, so all discussions could be kept confidential. But who is going to pay for that? We are no longer allowed to call out patient names in our office waiting room, because everyone hears the name. Isn't it getting ridiculous? Wouldn't the time, effort, and money have been better spent on something useful, like healthcare and education?

Our ethical code already includes protecting confidential information. When a company or the IRS is hacked, and our sensitive information stolen, they just say "sorry." Yet physicians are held to the highest standard and per patient fines. We need to use some common sense when new rules get enacted. Unfortunately, it seems that common sense isn't common.

15.1   HIPPA's Effect on Research

HIPPA rules have negatively affected the ability to perform research. How can a retrospective chart review be performed if the prior patients did not give their approval? Or prospectively calling patients for follow-up information?

Research study's informed consents must now include a section on how the patient's sensitive data will be protected.

A University of Michigan study concluded that there was a decrease from 96% to 34% in the proportion of heart attack victims completing follow-up studies resulting from the HIPPA rule.

Another study, detailing the effects of HIPAA on recruitment for a study on cancer prevention, demonstrated that

HIPAA-mandated changes led to a 73% decrease in patient accrual, a tripling of time spent recruiting patients, and a tripling of mean recruitment costs.

Suggested Reading

Armstrong D, Kline-Rogers E, Jani S, Goldman E, et al. Potential impact of the HIPAA privacy rule on data collection in a registry of patients with acute coronary syndrome. Arch Intern Med. 2005;165(10):1125–9.https://doi.org/10.1001/archinte.165.10.1125. PMID 15911725.

Wolf M, Bennett C. Local perspective of the impact of the HIPAA privacy rule on research. Cancer. 2006;106(2):474–9. https://doi.org/10.1002/cncr.21599. PMID 16342254.

Chapter 16
Political Interference

The recent overturning of Roe V. Wade (Dobbs decision) has again placed physicians in the crosshairs. Depending on which state you live in, you may be subject to fines and prison for violating the politician's interpretation of the laws, that themselves frequently don't even understand. You have a choice, leave the state, do not practice obstetrics, or continue to do what your ethics tell you to do and lie if you need to justify your actions.

Evidence of political influence was instrumental in the peripatetic COVID-19 response depending on which state you were in; State Surgeon Generals who did not believe in vaccines, or masking, and attacks on reputable scientists.

In Florida, I as a physician, am not allowed to ask a patient if they have guns in the house. As a condition of licensure, though I am an ophthalmologist, I also must pay an annual $250.00 for babies injured during birth and $5.00 for investigation of unlicensed practitioners.

The 1999 Dickey Amendment limited federal funding for gun violence research. The Centers for Disease Control and Prevention (CDC) Behavioral risk Factor Surveillance System collects data on seatbelt use and fruit juice consumption, but not access to guns. In 2019, Congress finally appropriated $25 million for gun violence research so hopefully there will now be research on gun violence and its prevention.

© The Author(s), under exclusive license to Springer Nature Switzerland AG 2023
J. N. Weiss, *Physician Crisis*,
https://doi.org/10.1007/978-3-031-27979-9_16

People without medical training and in some cases without intelligence or ethics, who on the basis of their own self-interest, and not that of your patient, are telling you how to practice medicine. The beginning of authoritarianism is the restriction of people's rights.

16.1   Corruptions Perceptions Index (CPI)

The CPI ranks countries "by their perceived levels of public sector corruption, as determined by expert assessments and opinion surveys" and has been published annually by Transparency International since 1995 (Table 16.1).

The U.S. is ranked #27, in a tie with Chile.

TABLE 16.1 Rankings

Legend:

Scores	Perceived as less corrupt				Perceived as more corrupt				
	89–90	79–80	69–60	59–50	49–40	39–30	29–20	19–10	9–0

2012–2021

Corruption Perceptions Index table

#	Nation or Territory	2021[a] Score	2021 Δ	2020[b] Score	2019[c] Score	2019 Δ	2018[d] Score	2018 Δ	2017[e] Score	2017 Δ	2016[f] Score	2016 Δ	2015[g] Score	2015 Δ	2014[h] Score	2014 Δ	2013[i] Score	2013 Δ	2012[j] Score	2012 Δ
1	Denmark	88	—	88	87	◀1	88	▶1	88	—	90	▶2	91	▶1	92	▶1	91	◀1	90	◀1
1	New Zealand	88	—	88	87	◀1	87	—	89	▶2	90	▶1	91	▶1	91	—	91	—	90	◀1
1	Finland	88	◀3	85	86	▶1	85	◀1	85	—	89	▶4	90	▶1	89	◀1	89	—	90	▶1
4	Singapore	85	—	85	85	—	85	—	84	◀1	84	—	85	▶1	84	◀1	86	▶2	87	▶1
4	Sweden	85	—	85	85	—	85	—	84	◀1	88	▶4	89	▶1	87	◀2	89	▶2	88	◀1
4	Norway	85	◀1	84	84	—	84	—	85	▶1	85	—	87	▶2	86	◀1	86	—	85	◀1

(continued)

TABLE 16.1 (continued)

#	Nation or Territory	2012 Score	2012 ▲	2013 Score	2013 ▲	2014 Score	2014 ▲	2015 Score	2015 ▲	2016 Score	2016 ▲	2017 Score	2017 ▲	2018 Score	2018 ▲	2019 Score	2019 ▲	2020 Score	2021 ▲	2021 Score
7	Switzerland	86	▶1	85	◀	86	|	86	|	86	▶1	85	|	85	|	85	|	85	▶1	84
8	Netherlands	84	▶1	83	|	83	◀4	87	▶4	83	▶1	82	|	82	|	82	|	82	|	82
10	Germany	79	▶1	78	◀	79	◀2	81	|	81	|	81	▶1	80	|	80	|	80	|	80
9	Luxembourg	80	|	80	◀1	82	▶1	81	|	81	◀1	82	▶1	81	▶1	80	|	80	◀1	81
18	Austria	85	▶4	81	▶1	80	▶1	79	|	79	▶2	77	|	77	|	77	|	77	▶4	73
13	Canada	84	▶3	81	|	81	◀2	83	▶1	82	|	82	▶1	81	▶4	77	|	77	▶3	74
12	Hong Kong	77	▶2	75	▶1	74	◀1	75	◀2	77	|	77	▶1	76	|	76	◀1	77	▶1	76
11	United Kingdom	74	◀2	76	◀2	78	◀3	81	|	81	◀1	82	▶2	80	▶3	77	|	77	◀1	78
13	Austria	69	|	69	◀3	72	◀4	76	▶1	75	|	75	◀1	76	◀1	77	▶1	76	▶2	74
18	Belgium	75	|	75	◀1	76	◀1	77	|	77	▶2	75	|	75	|	75	◀1	76	▶3	73

#	Nation or Territory	2021 Score	2021 ▲	2020 Score	2019 Score	2019 ▲	2018 Score	2018 ▲	2017 Score	2017 ▲	2016 Score	2016 ▲	2015 Score	2015 ▲	2014 Score	2014 ▲	2013 Score	2013 ▲	2012 Score	2012 ▲
13	Estonia	74	►1	75	74	◄1	73	◄1	71	◄2	70	◄1	70	|	69	◄1	68	◄1	64	◄4
13	Iceland	74	►1	75	78	►3	76	◄2	77	►1	78	►1	79	►1	79	|	78	◄1	82	►4
18	Japan	73	►1	74	73	◄1	73	|	73	|	72	◄1	75	►3	76	►1	74	◄2	74	|
13	Ireland	74	◄2	72	74	►2	73	◄1	74	►1	73	◄1	75	►2	74	◄1	72	◄2	69	◄3
24	United Arab Emirates	69	►2	71	71	|	70	◄1	71	►1	66	◄5	70	►4	70	|	69	◄1	68	◄1
18	Uruguay	73	◄2	71	71	|	70	◄1	70	|	71	►1	74	►3	73	◄1	73	|	72	◄1
22	France	71	◄1	69	69	|	72	►3	70	◄2	69	◄1	70	►1	69	◄1	71	►2	71	|
25	Bhutan	68	|	68	68	|	68	|	67	◄1	65	◄2	65	|	65	|	63	◄2	63	|
27	Chile	67	|	67	67	|	67	|	67	|	66	◄1	70	►4	73	►3	71	◄2	72	►1
27	United States	67	|	67	69	►2	71	►2	75	►4	74	◄1	76	►2	74	◄2	73	◄1		|

Suggested Reading

Cahan E. Lawsuits, reimbursement, and liability insurance-facing the ralities of a post-Roe era. JAMA. 2022;328(6):515–7.

Podobnik B, Shao J, Njavro D, et al. Influence of corruption on economic growth rate and foreign investment. Eur Phys J B. 2008;63(4):547. https://doi.org/10.1140/epjb/e2008.

Shao J, Ivanov PC, Podobnik B, Stanley HE. Quantitative relations between corruption and economic factors. Eur Phys J B. 2007;56(2):157. https://doi.org/10.1140/epjb/e2007-00098-2.

Wikiwand. Corruption perceptions index (latest). Transparency international. 2022. Accessed 25 Jan 2022.

Wilhelm PG. International validation of the corruption perceptions index: implications for business ethics and entrepreneurship education. J Bus Ethics. 2002;35(3):177–89. https://doi.org/10.1023/A:1013882225402.

Chapter 17
Miscellaneous — Other Thoughts

I rented office space on the for-profit hospital campus for almost 29 years. During that time, I never missed a rent payment. When I finally decided to close my office, my lease was set to expire on October 31. I asked for an extension to December 31, as I had found a potential buyer for my practice. The rental agent, hopeful that he would have a new rent paying tenant, confirmed that they would hold the rent constant until the end of the year, without the signing of a new lease. The deal concluded, but the purchaser decided to take my charts and equipment and move elsewhere. My office was emptied by the first week of December. I paid the entire November and December rent.

In March the following year, I received a bill for an additional $800 for "rent." They had apparently retrospectively increased my rental amount for November and December. I called the rental agent who said this came from "corporate." There was no number for the corporate office but with some sleuthing I found one. I left multiple messages but no one returned my call.

A month later I received a letter from an attorney demanding the $800 plus a $2000 attorney fee. I telephoned the attorney and explained what had happened. He said this came from "corporate." I told him I had a deal with the rental agent, I had actually left the premises 3 weeks early and was not paying anything additional. The attorney filed a lawsuit against me, and now the demand was for $16,000, the extra $15,000 was for his legal fees.

The lawyer's office was 4 h north of me, and though he could have attended the court hearing remotely, he chose to drive to Broward County and charge for the time. Even the Judge pointed out that he didn't need to appear in person at the hearing.

Their lawyer had sent lots of information requests. I answered them myself. They wanted me to get an attorney, but I represented myself. In listening to my explanation to the Judge, I realized how right I sounded and how stupid the hospital attorney sounded. They never expected me to go to court, but to cave and pay them their extortion money.

I won the case. When I returned to the doctor's dining room the physicians congratulated me and slapped me on the back. The administrators refused to look at me, it was the first time they had ever lost. All the other doctors, when threatened, had backed down. I had set a dangerous precedent. I didn't cave. I fought back, and won.

The descent of physician respect to the low level we are at now began when they started calling us "Providers." The first step in denigrating a group is to destroy their self-esteem. History is replete with examples. Physicians should have rebelled then, but we accepted it. After all, even the most corrupt politician or Judge is still called by their correct title.

It is said that getting physicians to agree on anything is like "herding cats." And the "other side" knows this. They also know that we are committed to patient care, and can use our own ethics and humanity against us. And since the public thinks all physicians are making millions, any fight for increased reimbursement with the insurance companies will fall on the deaf ears of the public.

When I was in medical school, one of my attendings had holes in the soles of his shoes. This was to show us that he didn't care about himself, only his patients. That attitude has now brought us to the present time. We care about our patients, but we must also care about ourselves, because no one else does.

Another way to denigrate us is to say everyone is "equal." When my friends asked the scrub technician for a critical instrument in the operating room, or a floor secretary for laboratory work, and their response was it wasn't their job, my friends got upset. The scrub nurse, and the secretary reported these physicians to administration, and both doctors were forced to take a month long anger management class. No mention was made as to why the instrument or laboratory work was missing, or whose job it was to ensure that the required items were there as both affected patient care. We are only the "captain of the ship," when there is a lawsuit, not for anything else.

When one of the physicians was killed in an accident, at the next hospital meeting, the first thing the administrator said was that they had spent a lot of money on the instruments they bought him. Such compassion.

Another issue is "off-label" use of medications, devices, and procedures. I gave the example of the gas retinal specialists used for 20 years before it was FDA approved. The price went from $70 to $1500 just for a sticker on the exact same gas cannister. Since the cost for FDA approval is so high, drugs and devices that are inexpensive, or with a limited market are seldom approved, even when they are much better and safer than existing "approved" products.

There was a chemical approved in Europe which made peeling the internal limiting membrane from the retina much safer. But it wasn't approved in the U.S. Retinal specialists used other less safe and less efficacious methods to perform the surgery, or paid compounding pharmacies to mix the drug for them. The patients suffered. Years later, the company spent the money and the same drug was finally approved. Like the gas, it was the same item we used for years without incident, but it now was "approved," and became expensive. It was always "approved" by the physicians using it.

Companies are not allowed to speak about anything that is "off-label," or not "approved" even when it clearly benefits the patient. But isn't this how doctors learn? If a treatment doesn't work it is discarded through the practice of medicine.

The FDA is not supposed to be practicing medicine, but by its regulations, it is, similar to the "activist" Judges who by their rulings are making, not enforcing laws.

I left academics in Boston when it ceased to be academics. Seeing patients and performing surgery made money. Though my grant paid for 2 days of my time, patients were scheduled 5 days per week. And they were double and sometimes triple booked in the same time spot. The joke was for the patient to bring a copy of "War and Peace." But it wasn't funny. Patients waited unnecessarily for hours, just so the institution could make more money.

I needed to present to the Grant Committee, which met infrequently, with any purchase requests from my grant. Then the institution increased their overhead to 100%, which made my grant applications non-competitive in terms of the money I was asking for. Nowadays, the academics perform drug studies dictated by, and paid for, by pharmaceutical companies. There is little truly novel, beneficial research being done.

A recent article in nature confirms that despite the tremendous increase in the number of published papers and patents, the percent of truly novel disruptive innovation has declined. From 1980 to 2010, there has been a 91.5% decrease in the number of drug and medical patents. More people are performing their work in narrower avenues and therefore not producing groundbreaking work. The "Cancer Moonshot" of the National Cancer Institute is a potential response to this problem.

There are multiple explanations for the decrease. Inventors are patenting improvements to their existing patents in order to retain their licensing rights. Funding institutions favor conservative and guaranteed results, rather than "moonshots." To obtain an NIH grant, half of the research has to already be completed. Non-academic physicians are excluded from receiving grants. Journals accept variations on earlier, more familiar work, rather than something truly new. And professional societies, funded by drug and device companies, protect their own interests. They support those companies that support them, and punish the individual innovator that doesn't send money to their own coffers.

Experimental psychologist, Adam Mastroianni of Columbia Business School has said, "If you wanted to design a system that prevents innovation, you'd probably come up with something similar to the way science works right now." He continued, "make scientists spend half their time asking for money. Don't publish anything until it has satisfied reviewer's whims. Exclude hobbyists, amateurs, and anyone with strange ideas. And most importantly, make the whole thing so competitive that everybody's terrified of taking any risk. That system will produce lots of papers, but little progress." Much like the interminable movie sequels and absence of original works.

Private funding for research used to be the answer. Corporate funding, like Bell Labs, produced transistors, cellphones, and internet technology, have now vanished. Present day corporations are driven by their quarterly stock prices, not by long-term research, which may or may not be successful.

Those physicians contemplating research careers should bear this in mind.

Chapter 18
Possible Solutions

The U.S. healthcare system is the best in the world for some, and the worst for others. The U.S. spends the most per capita in the world, yet many people are uninsured, or underinsured. HMO's restrict care and patients suffer or die as a result. U.S. pharmaceutical prices are the highest in the world, though the drugs are manufactured by U.S. companies. 100 million Americans have health care debt, 1/3 of those due to a hospitalization.

The strong lobbies and large amounts of money at stake restrict the ability of truly across the board meaningful reform. The government is good at spending money, politicians rarely bite the hand the feeds them. There is no political consensus whether healthcare is a right or a privilege.

What is the answer? Physicians are under tremendous stress. The system is designed to take advantage of us. With more physicians becoming hospital employees, perhaps in the distant future, we will be unionized, much like the nurses have already done. The government will push back on physician unionization because they are part of the problem and have a vested interest in keeping physicians under their thumb and without a voice or power. There are few munificent CEO's who give large bonuses to valued employees or pay for children's college tuitions. That is why, when it happens, it makes national news.

© The Author(s), under exclusive license to Springer Nature   95
Switzerland AG 2023
J. N. Weiss, *Physician Crisis*,
https://doi.org/10.1007/978-3-031-27979-9_18

The reality is that healthcare is a business, despite our noble feelings, and that when care is provided at the lowest price, the entity providing the care makes more money. Since they make the definition of "quality" they can justify anything. We as physicians, know, that their definition of quality is different than ours.

A local hospital advertised that they were in the "top 10% of hospitals in the nation." I looked into this claim and found it was for medical record completion, not patient care. Without unionization, we are at the mercy of everyone. Our professional organizations are toothless tigers, they cannot force change. In large measure they are run by physicians without any true business experience. Look to the Teamsters for the ability to force change.

Things could improve when important people are impacted. The number of hours worked by residents in New York City were reduced when the daughter of a prominent person died at a hospital because the resident taking care of her was overworked and exhausted. That's what it took, not years of complaining.

The nature of the practice of medicine is stressful. How do you minimize the added stresses of insurance companies, the government, liability, EMR, hospital administration, etc.?

It all depends on what you want out of life. If you have no interest in business, don't need or care about making a lot of money, and just want to practice medicine, there are several routes open to you.

1. Volunteer work, i.e., doctors without borders.
2. Become an employee of an organization working in an underserved community.
3. Open your own practice and take no insurance, cash only. You will not be subject to the myriad of changing regulations, unfunded mandates, collection difficulties, and mandatory EMR adoption.
4. Move to another country and practice there. I have done volunteer work in the South Pacific and China and that has been among my most memorable experiences practicing medicine. The patients were extremely appreciative, and

the documentation was only for the patient benefit, not to justify my work to an insurance company or to protect myself from liability, or perform an unfunded mandate to satisfy a meaningless government directive written by someone with no concept of medical practice.

5. Try locum tenens to get a feel for the geographical area you wish to work. This gives you the flexibility in managing your own schedule, the ability to interact and learn from many different providers, to isolate yourself from the bureaucracy and politics of permanently working in an institution, and to travel. If you're unhappy, you can always leave and go somewhere else.

Since the beginning of the COVID-19 pandemic, 46% of physicians have changed jobs, a 2022 CHG Healthcare survey found. Almost half of the respondents quit their jobs in order to reduce stress and gain control over their lives.

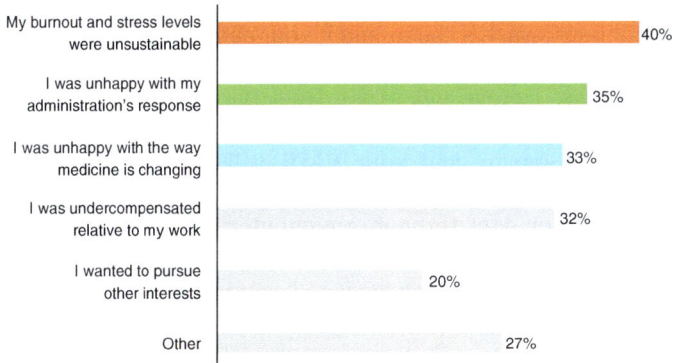

If you want to gain experience, work for a for-profit hospital chain for 2 years. You will learn, find the experience unfavorable, and then leave to work somewhere else. My friend was Chief of Pathology at a very large for-profit hospital chain. After almost 20 years working for them, and about to receive his pension, a friend of his telephoned him to say that the Hospital was running an ad for his job. He came in on a Monday, 6 months before retirement, was fired, and escorted by security to the parking lot. A similar event happened to the Chief Nurse who was about to retire and receive her pension. Don't think your loyalty to them will pay off. It isn't reciprocated.

A non-profit hospital chain may be better. But remember, you serve at the whim of the management, whomever that may be. New managers and administrations have different ideas.

The new administrator at a for-profit hospital wanted a surgeon to call his patients clients or guests, not patients. He refused and was fired. Another physician, employed by the hospital, was asked to narrate a commercial advertising the great benefits of being a hospital employee. He refused, and though being on staff for more than 20 years, but having sold his practice to the hospital 2 years earlier, was fired.

If you are in solo practice, you don't need EMR. Paper is much faster and easier. You can scan the paper into your computer so it can be accessed at home in case the patient telephones you. It's cheap, and if your pen runs out of ink you can get another. You aren't subjected to an initial expensive cost, future increasingly expensive service contracts, and the fear that your company may go bankrupt or be purchased by another company and your EMR will no longer be supported. Hacking and the resulting HIPPA violations, losing electricity, or data through a computer problem, are of no concern.

Another potential avenue is to become the "world expert" in a particular condition, disease, or treatment. Then you can be on your own. Of course, your jealous colleagues and Academic Medicine and your professional Academy will attack you because they aren't part of your success. Just expect that to happen. Physicians are jealous and ego driven, they seldom revel in the success of others.

Another alternative is to work for a large single or multi-specialty group. But you may encounter problems if it is owned by a private equity group, and not by the physicians. You may have a future there, but you will definitely have to deal with EMR and the potential fickleness of administration.

EMR will get better. It will become more intuitive, and physicians will have their own preloaded orders so they don't have to spend so much time clicking on things. The question is, do you want to be dealing with a system where you spend 2 h entering data for each 1 h of work now?

You should try to avoid dealing with insurance companies. I already alluded to some of my experiences dealing with them. Of note, years ago, Blue Cross was found to be throwing out physician claims in the garbage. They apologized, nothing more.

When I complained to the Florida Insurance Board that Humana wasn't paying me, they referred me to a for-profit company to handle my claim. The Head of the Florida Insurance Board later went to work for an insurance company.

How can ants protect themselves from the whim of elephants? They stay away from them.

Chapter 19
Summary

1. Try to minimize unnecessary stress.
2. Remember, you are a member of a noble profession.
3. Make conscious decisions about the meetings you attend and those you don't.
4. Don't waste your time on non-worthwhile hospital activities—meetings, committees, especially if they have no power and are just rubber stamps for administration.
5. Don't deal with organizations that are difficult to deal with or who aren't dealing fairly with you.
6. If you are unhappy in your present working situation, change it.
7. The past is over, the present is now, and don't worry about the future, create it.
8. Honest people interpret rules the way they were intended. People lacking integrity hide behind the commas in any agreement. A contract can be 120 pages long, but it is the integrity of the person signing the document that truly determines whether it will honored.
9. And if you are so depressed and having suicidal thoughts, get help. There is no stigma in seeking help and it can save your life.

© The Author(s), under exclusive license to Springer Nature   101
Switzerland AG 2023
J. N. Weiss, *Physician Crisis*,
https://doi.org/10.1007/978-3-031-27979-9_19

Chapter 20
This May Save Your Life

As physicians, we are all aware of medical errors. In Florida, as a condition of licensure, we must take a "Medical Errors" course every 2 years. The course is always the same.

The "errors" are divided into different types, much like in baseball, but there is nothing we can do about them. We have no power. The major problem leading to medical errors is the lack of competent staffing, both nursing and physician. Physicians and nurses are overworked and stressed by the endless bureaucracy and lack of respect. Here are some examples of unfortunately true stories:

1. A physician was admitted to a famous Boston teaching hospital for a broken hip. His treating physician forgot to put him on a blood thinner. His last act was to call his wife telling her about his sense of impending death. This emotion is seen in patients with pulmonary embolism. He called for help and no one came. He developed a pulmonary embolism and died.
2. An elderly patient called for a nurse so she could go to the bathroom. No one came. She tried to get out of bed to go to the bathroom. She fell and was injured.
3. A physician was receiving intravenous antibiotics as treatment for diverticulitis. The nurse checked his identification, and the bar code on the intravenous bag, and proceeded to hang the wrong intravenous bag. The physician patient saw

© The Author(s), under exclusive license to Springer Nature Switzerland AG 2023
J. N. Weiss, *Physician Crisis*,
https://doi.org/10.1007/978-3-031-27979-9_20

the mistake and it was corrected. She was the only medication night nurse for an entire wing of patients and was exhausted.

4. A physician chose the best surgeon to perform a robotic repair of his diverticulitis. He also chose the best anesthesiologist at the hospital. He didn't realize that a urologist would be called to cannulate his ureters. A urologist he didn't know came late to the operating room and promptly ruptured both his ureters. He spent 10 days (as compared to the 3 days for a routine diverticulitis repair) in the hospital to recover.

5. Frequently, the scrub nurse in the operating room has no experience. Equipment is lost or broken. The surgeon must spend time making certain that all the necessary instruments and medications are available. Many times they are not, and more physician time is wasted.

6. Splints were fashioned for a child in the ICU. The splints were not cooled before being placed on the child and both arms were burned, resulting in scars. I reviewed the chart after discharge, the notes were re-written and the chart sanitized.

I know many more of these types of incidents. None of these incidents was ever reported. I am certain that you know of many more.

Unlike an aviation accident which the FAA looks for a solution, reporting a medical incident only looks to blame someone and may result in a lawsuit. Therefore, problems are swept under the rug.

My point is, if you are ever hospitalized, depending on the reason, you should have a physician advocate watching over you. Do not trust the support staff. They may be poorly trained, tired, and overworked. Try to control which physicians are treating you. Hopefully they will watch and keep your best interests at heart. Hospitals save money on staffing, many of the supposed "certifications" are not evidence of competence. If a hospital is hiring the least number of workers, at the lowest cost, you cannot expect competent service. "Murphy's Law" also applies to physician patients.

Chapter 21
Conclusion

It is my hope that the information presented in this book will guide you into being more satisfied and hopefully happier in our most noble of professions. Knowledge is power and with information you can make the appropriate decisions to respond to the ever-present challenges we as physicians face daily. I wish you the best of luck.

J. N. Weiss, *Physician Crisis*,
https://doi.org/10.1007/978-3-031-27979-9_21

Index

© The Editor(s) (if applicable) and The Author(s), under
exclusive license to Springer Nature Switzerland AG 2023
J. N. Weiss, *Physician Crisis*,
https://doi.org/10.1007/978-3-031-27979-9